Hot Mess Express is a humorous, inspiring story of surviving menopause, with detailed health information wrapped in Friscea's personal story. A handbook for all women facing the "pause."
—**Rachel Hauck**, *New York Times* best-selling author

Full of educational insights and tips about surviving and thriving through menopause, *Hot Mess Express* puts the reader at ease about The Change. Every woman should buy this book!
—**Michelle Medlock Adams**, best-selling author, award-winning journalist, author of *Paws-itive Inspirations* and *Aging Fabulously*

Authentic. Raw. Real. You will experience these emotional narratives on most pages of *Hot Mess Express* as Sally Friscea offers you a way to move forward despite the messiness of menopause. And not to be left out, just the right amount of humor, giving us a moment to nod our heads in agreement and giggle with understanding as only "those who know" can. *Hot Mess Express* provides a breath of hope for the woman who is ready to grab midlife by it's belly fat and move forward into a season of happily ever after the night sweats!
—**Linda Goldfarb**, multi-award-winning author and podcaster, board-certified Christian life coach, LindaGoldfarb.com

A must-read! Sally Friscea employs her unique talents to connect with women during a significant, yet challenging period of life. Through personal accounts, remedies, humor, and more, *Hot Mess Express* will entertain and provide educational insight for the reader. I highly recommend this book for women and the men in their lives.
—**Irene Wintermyer**, author, certified health coach, physician assistant and hospital director (ret.)

No one warns you. Not your mother. Not your grandmother. Not your great-aunt Matilda. Barely your doctor. Oh, sure. There are hints. Insinuations. But no one spells it out one letter of the alphabet at a time. Until now. And with the humor only Sally Friscea could produce. Because if you gotta go through menopause, you may as well laugh.

Otherwise, you'll cry yourself silly. And we have to go through it. (It's part of the curse not mentioned in Genesis—that and chin hairs.) My only regret is that I didn't have this book twenty—no, thirty—years ago! So . . . read! Learn! Laugh!
—**Eva Marie Everson**, best-selling author, CEO Word Weavers International

In *Hot Mess Express*, Sally Friscea offers a candid, relatable, and often humorous take on navigating the roller coaster of menopause and hormonal changes. From hot flashes to mood swings, Friscea addresses every symptom with honesty and compassion, helping readers feel understood and supported. This book is a must-read for women experiencing hormonal chaos. It's an empowering guide to reclaiming your health, well-being, and sense of self.
—**Susan Neal**, RN, MBA, MHS, author of *12 Ways to Age Gracefully*

I really appreciate author Sally Friscea for sharing her menopause experiences with humor along with the treatments. Be prepared to laugh as you read through all the chapters. And, truly, laughter is the best medicine.
—**Erica Ross**, registered nurse

HOT MESS
EXPRESS

A HUMOROUS *and* **PRACTICAL
SURVIVAL GUIDE** *for* **MENOPAUSE**

SALLY FRISCEA

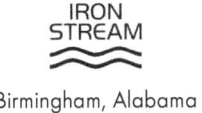

Birmingham, Alabama

Hot Mess Express

Iron Stream
An imprint of Iron Stream Media
100 Missionary Ridge
Birmingham, AL 35242
IronStreamMedia.com

Copyright © 2025 by Sally Friscea

All rights reserved. No part of this publication may be reproduced, stored in a retrieval system. or transmitted in any form or by any means—electronic, mechanical, photocopying, recording, or otherwise—without the prior written permission of the publisher.

Iron Steam Media serves its authors as they express their views, which may not express the views of the publisher.

Scripture quotations are taken from the World English Bible in the public domain.

Cover design by twolineSTUDIO.com

Library of Congress Control Number: 2024940857

ISBN: 978-1-56309-749-2 (paperback)
ISBN: 978-1-56309-751-5 (ebook)

1 2 3 4 5—29 28 27 26 25

DISCLAIMER: All content and information in this book is for informational and educational purposes only, does not constitute medical advice, and does not establish any kind of patient-client relationship by your reading of this book. Always seek the advice of your physician or other qualified health care provider with any questions you may have regarding a medical condition or treatment and before undertaking a new health care regimen, and never disregard professional medical advice or delay in seeking it because of something you read in this book.

To my husband, Dean,

whose bravery includes joining his life to mine in the middle of menopause and who also must have been so completely bored with life that he married me, presumably for his daily entertainment.

You're welcome.

I am in awe of your patience with others, including me— I know I can be a lot, but not as much as my brother.

Therefore we don't faint, but though our outward person is decaying, yet our inward person is renewed day by day.

—2 Corinthians 4:16

CONTENTS

The Warning. xi
1. How I Got Here 1
2. Estrogen Overload 7
3. What Are We Talking About?. 17
4. Insomnia. 23
5. Hormonal Rage and Mood Swings 51
6. Hot Flashes and Night Sweats 61
7. Hair. 69
8. Skin 87
9. Nails 107
10. Eyes 117
11. Inner Ear. 129
12. Mouth 133
13. Nose 143
14. Muscle Tone 151
15. Metabolism and Weight Gain. 169
16. Digestive Issues 179
17. Joints 187
18. Bones. 199
19. Healing 205
20. The Brain 209
21. Dehydration 217
22. What Is *Diet*?. 223
Summary. 233
Acknowledgments. 239
Notes 241

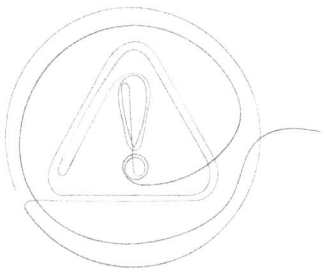

THE WARNING

If you survive your youthful indiscretions, accidents, or any number of unspeakable medical issues, you will get old. Ignorance is bliss. If you've picked up this book and you're still in your twenties or younger, skip to the last section of chapter 2, "Estrogen Overload." Heed the warning, get the baseline hormone test, and guard the results with your life. Then, place this book on your nightstand for a decade. Live in your ignorance. Enjoy your youth without a sense of impending doom.

THE FINE PRINT

Because I'm not a doctor, I suggest you see your doctor for any tests or diagnoses. But I intend to give you a heads-up about what you're experiencing. It might simply be a normal part of aging, not a life-threatening malady.

CHAPTER 1

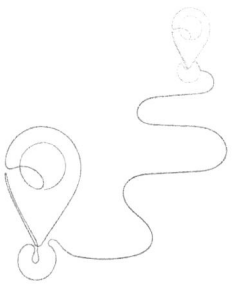

HOW I GOT HERE

Thyroid? Muscular Dystrophy? Cancer?

For five long years, I wondered what horrific disease befell me. A gazillion small things started to go wrong with me, but I couldn't connect them. Death of a thousand cuts. I didn't dare speak the words out loud for fear of a "negative confession" or "self-fulfilling prophecy" bringing into being what might not have otherwise happened; the mind is powerful and can convince the body to manifest what otherwise wasn't an actual medical condition previously.

No one warned me about the first subtle changes I faced during perimenopause, the stage before menopause when you transition from regular menstruations to sporadic periods.

Occasionally I'd heard an older person say, "Getting old is not for sissies." But no real information about the physical or mental changes followed that declaration.

Don't ask, don't tell.

No one I knew talked about it, and I didn't ask. I didn't know what to ask. I didn't associate the changes with anything in particular—a random cluster of unassociated symptoms. Mostly, I didn't pay attention until my body screamed for my attention.

Every day is a new adventure in how my body will betray me.

I Used to Be Cool

I wasn't just a legend in my own mind. I was actually cool—an eighties new-wave club girl and fashion-forward to the point that my fashion merchandising college professor picked on me. She didn't like my half-shaved head or my sneakers—green Chuck Taylors. I admit the second-hand store polyester bowling shirt with the name *Bill* stitched on the chest might have been a tad too much. But it ranked as hip, hot, trend-setting—black and white with a gray diamond design. And I was cool, just underappreciated in 1980s Louisiana.

Then, slowly, almost unnoticeably, my body, energy, mind, and even my tastes in food and clothes changed. They all "matured."

My clothing tastes had faded from cutting-edge and punk in my late teens and early twenties to blending in more at church and general society. I considered it better to overdress for any occasion than underdress.

My awareness of fashion trends didn't help as a general fashion malaise overtook me in my forties.

In 2010, during the Great Recession, my mother and I moved in together to save money after I'd had a couple of steep pay cuts. As an extrovert, I welcomed the company. Still single in my forties, I'd finally realized why the older single ladies no longer attended the church's singles group, a constant reminder of an unmarried status. Gradually, I joined their ranks. Living alone gave me too much time to ponder my lingering, lonely situation, and I'd started feeling sorry for myself. I'd grown slightly disheartened. Therefore, Mom and I combined households for both companionship and finances.

How I Got Here

On weekends, we would shop together. One time, I held up a shirt, "Mom, is this top cute? I can't tell anymore." I'd become too tired and too discouraged to care anymore.

She said yes, and I purchased it. This continued for six years until I had a closet full of clothes I'd picked out with my mother. Age-appropriate clothes but not youthful styles—clothes I'd noticed on the older ladies at church. It had been ten years since I'd ventured into a junior's section of a department store, though I was small enough, and I enjoyed the cheaper prices. No longer hip enough to bother, I'd probably aged out long ago; somewhere along the way, I'd struggled to stay in style and not succumb to the increased desire for comfort.

Subsequently, I'd reverted to my childhood years when my mother picked out my clothes.

People almost always guessed me to be much younger than my age until then. My love language is affirmation, so I enjoyed thirty years of compliments on my youthful looks. At eighteen, I looked twelve. At thirty, twenty. Even at forty, I'd been mistaken for late twenties now and again. But after the first five years of sleep deprivation, I was no longer getting mistaken as a decade-plus younger. My wardrobe aged with my face, but I'd had no idea to what extent. After a decade of crickets, I craved a little flattery.

In the summer of 2016, at the age of forty-eight, I met a man. We had no previous marriages and no children. I observed him at church for a while and wondered how he remained single all these years. I waited for the reason to present itself, but it didn't. He told me he, too, looked for the crazy factor. He believed all women were crazy to some extent.

We had lunches together after Sunday church services through the fall. Then, in January, Dean finally asked me out on a proper date. Months later, when I felt completely comfortable with him, I asked, "How old did you think I was when we first met?" When he hesitated, I told him, "There's no wrong answer." A softball question, an easy homerun hit for him. Time passed as I waited patiently.

He finally eked out, "Sixty?"

My head felt light. Stars speckled my vision.

Did my ears deceive me? "What?"

His eyes widened. Rattled in his tone, Dean replied, "You said there was no wrong answer."

Alas, a wrong answer. "Why did you guess me a decade older than you?"

He said, "Well, it's all the burkas and turtlenecks you wear."

An Afghani-blue burka hung in my closet—for posterity, a piece of history. I'd found it years before while perusing exotic wedding dresses online. And I had two turtlenecks for the short Florida winters, but he'd never seen any of those items. He referred to the age-appropriate tunics I favored. They're the long, comfortable three-quarter sleeve shirts. They usually cover the rump, so you don't have to worry about panty lines—increasingly more important when even my stretch jeans became too tight.

I modeled a turtleneck for Dean at church the next weekend to make a point. Afterward, we went out for lunch with a group who'd chosen to eat outside in the eighty-five-degree weather. I pushed up the sleeves and pulled at the neckline. I paid dearly for that joke.

During one tug, he teased. "That'll teach you to spite me."

We married anyway, and we've been laughing at each other and ourselves ever since. A pastor at a previous church told my mother, "She's going to have to marry a strong man." He wasn't wrong. And I did.

That same year, I'd dropped by a housewarming party for one of my brother's friends. I stood beside a twentysomething guy in our group conversation. Since he didn't know me, I asked him to guess my age and gave him the same caveat I'd given Dean about no wrong answer. My brother, Joe, has always looked younger, too,

How I Got Here

so I figured I had him for sure, like the carnival barker at the Guess Your Age booth during my thirties who'd undershot by a decade.

But no. "Forty-eight?" Dead on.

What was happening?

Probably because my mouth hung open, he offered, "Don't worry about it, I'm a bartender. It's my job to know."

The reasonable answer did nothing for my ego. People always guessed me as younger, and I banked on this trend continuing into my twilight years.

Age caught up with me like a zombie horde—you might be able to stay ahead of it for a while, but eventually, you tire out, and it overtakes you. Aging affects every aspect of your life, with most of the effects coming from hormonal changes. That is why they call it The Change.

Men go through it too. Don't let them tell you they don't. It is evidenced by the gradual decrease in testosterone, which leads to lower metabolism, weight gain, lower libido, and so on. Besides, there are far too many Corvettes and old muscle cars sold to men between the ages of fifty and sixty for that not to be true.

These purchases may have more to do with the stage of life when they finally have enough money to acquire some of those toys they've wanted since high school. But, if you're married and all your husband does is buy an expensive toy during his midlife crisis, consider yourself blessed.

Over the years, I took copious mental notes on crazy stories for when, if ever, I married. Those included stories of affairs, divorces, and homosexual "coming out" announcements, and now I'm getting wind of people questioning their gender at older ages. Yes, these things happen at all ages, but they seem to cluster around hormonal life changes. And at both ends—adolescence and midlife crisis ages.

Simply an expensive toy? Absolutely.

Dodged that bullet.

CHAPTER 2

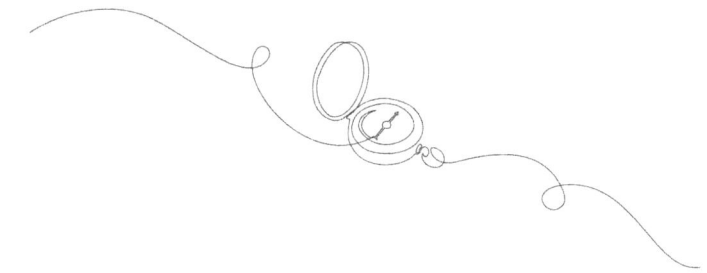

ESTROGEN OVERLOAD

In the Beginning

What is going on?

Raging hormones can make you feel like you're going crazy or that you're alone in this. But you're not. Like growing up, everybody changes. It simply affects some more than others and in different ways.

As stated previously, I'm one of the unfortunate ones who tended toward the extremes. Hormones got me coming and going. Nobody ever talked about it, including me. I started menstruating at a normal age—if not a little later than average—at thirteen. But instead of having three- to five-day periods, mine were often seven to eight and particularly heavy for the three middle days.

One of those first heavy days happened during ninth grade. I sat in class wearing lime-green pants. I raised my hand too late. I went from fine during the previous hour's bathroom check to pure panic.

It may have been the first, but it was not the only time menstruation mishaps embarrassed me. A multitude of such occasions plagued me as if, somehow, I could not learn to accept the changes happening in my body.

My sister, a mere eighteen months older and only a grade ahead, used tampons. I figured what worked for her must work for me too. I learned the hard way for most things, with this being one of the hardest. After a user-error mishap when a too-dry tampon almost refused to come out, I steered clear of the cotton rascals for years.

The generation behind me had to put up with belts on pads. Grandma spoke of scraps of material used to catch the flow. Instead, I endured pads. Sanitary napkins, a name far from the truth. But it felt like I wore a Barbie doll bed in my days-of-the-week underwear. My smaller body could barely keep up with my monthly period.

Throughout my life, this cyclic blood loss has affected me in myriad ways. For example, it compromised my habit of donating blood for three reasons. First, I would routinely fail the predonation iron test—the blood wouldn't sink in the test tube—eliminating my chance of donating. Second, I've always been a remarkable coagulator. I clot easily, making it hard for the blood to fill a bag before my body starts repairing the hole—the skin adheres to the needle, shutting down the process. Third, sometimes, they could not locate a suitable vein since I didn't get enough fluids. I later learned to drink extra water before donating or doctor-ordered tests. After one gal at the blood bank wasted all five chances to find a vein, I determined to request the most experienced phlebotomist and asked for a butterfly needle.

After the Exam

Right after I turned forty, I got a running start on the aging process. I went from a seven- or eight-day menstrual period to more than eleven days. As it crept past two weeks, my concern flared.

Estrogen Overload

When I reached three weeks, I visited my gynecologist. Dr. I. tried to look at my uterus in the office, but it didn't hold water, so the scope wouldn't work. After the exam, she scheduled me for same-day surgery. The doctor explained that if she found something, she could do something about it immediately.

She asked, "Where are you with having children?"

"I haven't even started, but I'd like to keep the door open as long as possible in case God finally sends me a husband."

After I woke up, the doctor said, "You had a fibroid practically the size of your uterus, but we removed it." She turned toward my mother. "That's why it took more time. Sorry to worry you, Mom." She turned back to me. "We're having it tested, but I think it's benign. Take it easy for a couple of days."

"How big is a uterus?" I asked.

She held up her fist.

"That's a big fibroid."

She agreed. "But it's not uncommon. I used to practice in the Caribbean and saw a lot of these." She chuckled and left.

The fibroid test showed no cancer, and my periods returned to my usual seven to eight days of bloodletting. Studies are inconclusive as to the cause of uterine fibroid tumors, but higher estrogen levels are suspected.

Seven years later, the flow increased to twenty-plus days again. By then, we were fully into the Great Recession, and I'd lost my health insurance. I returned to the Veterans Administration (VA) on the Space Coast of Florida. They sent me to the new Orlando VA hospital to see a specialist.

"Where are you in family planning?" the new doctor asked.

"At forty-seven years old, I haven't even started yet, and I suppose I'd like to keep the door open if possible."

The doctor first addressed the excessive bleeding with an IUD (intrauterine device), which my body expelled within a couple of months and required extra tests to make sure the IUD hadn't dislodged somewhere into my body rather than a toilet. Then, he recommended an ablation to remove the lining of my uterus. After hearing that the odds would be less than 50 percent for success, I passed on the procedure.

After many tests and months of visits, I decided I'd had enough. "Take it all."

The gynecological expert explained the benefits of taking the uterus and fallopian tubes but leaving the ovaries. My risk of uterine and fallopian cancer would drop significantly. The remaining ovaries would continue to make hormones, meaning I wouldn't have to take hormone pills. That made a partial hysterectomy an easy answer.

And I wouldn't grow a beard.

He didn't say the last part. I interpreted it as such, but joining the circus wasn't an option.

As my life plans clashed with a twenty-year delay in getting married, I explained to him I didn't exactly hear a clock ticking for babies, but I also didn't want to slam the door shut prematurely . . . at forty-seven.

Bad timing. I'd never had the desire to have children and change diapers, see them off to school, or kiss them goodnight. My family took bets on plants and pets dying under my care. During the eighties, I had a button on my backpack of a woman waking from a nap, wondering if she'd left the baby on the bus. Totally me. I did want to be normal—get married, have kids, then spoil the grandkids—but more than that, I wanted whatever God wanted for me.

And yet I'd been standing on the rock of faith all those years, trusting that if I had children, God would fill my heart full of His love for them and give me what I needed when I felt inadequate to parent.

Estrogen Overload

God is able. I believe in the book of Isaiah, which says that he opens and closes the womb. I left the matter of having children in His hands.

My desire to be normal and have a husband with a statistical 2.3 children overwhelmed me. Yet it conflicted with the reality of my lack of desire to be pregnant and my advancing age. I pondered Mary, who got pregnant without a man. I wondered about Sarah, who finally conceived in her nineties. And I didn't forget about Elizabeth, who had John the Baptist well past her child-bearing years.

However, at that time, I only related to the woman with an issue of blood. I didn't want to die from loss of blood either. How I related to her, crying out to God and boldly touching the hem of Jesus's garment and instantly receiving her healing.

Yes, God is more than able.

Believing, I'd cried out for years for healing and had others pray with no instant outcome. Not even a slow, steady result. Only a progressive worsening.

Pregnancy isn't for all women. Some of us aren't physically able to do it, and then there's timing—I didn't plan to do motherhood on my own. I'd seen it go wrong many times. It's one thing to accidentally find yourself in that position, but it's quite another to purposefully choose it.

A partial hysterectomy screamed finality. And yet, bleeding to death did too.

Over the years, all the appointments, tests, and procedures left me exhausted—not simply because of low iron.

As I was ever the guinea pig, the gynecologist shared my pelvic exams with other professionals. The specialist asked me, "You don't mind if Doctor Jones stands in on this exam, do you? She's learning."

Yes, I do mind. Am I in Amsterdam's red-light district displaying my goods in a glass-front brothel?

"No," I replied, "the more the merrier." My sarcasm did not translate well. I didn't realize I had a choice at the VA to decline his request.

During the exam, the specialist told the training doctor. "Get way in there and see if you can find her cervix tilted to the side." Then he asked her, "Can you feel her enlarged uterus?" With one hand in me and the other on my abdomen, she felt around for what felt like minutes as her face showed uncertainty.

My pelvic ultrasound went much the same way. "Do you mind if Laura controls the vaginal wand? She's learning."

"No, why would I?" I replied. "Will there be a class of doctors making their way into my exam room shortly, as you see on television with the hospital shows?"

Deep inside, I cried, *Uncle!*

After years of sleeping on just-in-case towels, popping copious amounts of ibuprofen trying to keep the pain manageable, and throwing away numerous ruined clothing and undergarments, I conceded my loss and awaited the partial hysterectomy.

The specialist put me on a strong dose of birth control pills and sent me on my way while I waited for the VA to schedule my procedure. After two long months, I had an appointment for a presurgical evaluation in Tampa—only two short hours across to the other side of the state.

After two more months, another crowded exam room in the Tampa VA hospital, and numerous calls, they finally released me to the Choice program, which allows veterans who live far from a VA facility to obtain medical care from someone closer to home. A program representative called to tell me I had until the end of the year to find a private practice to do the procedure and any follow-up. That left me two months. I called and found someone in my county and made an appointment. I explained the time constraints.

Estrogen Overload

(Never mind this whole process was approaching a year and a half for a "life-saving surgery.")

They fit me into their schedule. Two weeks later, I arrived to more paperwork. A half-hour later, I turned in a small novel of forms. They showed me back to the exam room and presented me with a paper garment. "Opening at the front, please."

Breezy.

I endured another routinely uncomfortable exam. After I dressed, the nurse escorted me to the doctor's office. "Well, I'm getting ready to go on maternity leave and can't fit you in until February. How does that sound?"

"When I scheduled, I informed the front office that I'd have until the end of the year to get this taken care of." With a calm demeanor, I fumed inside.

"If you can't wait, you can schedule with another doctor in the office."

And waste a month waiting for another appointment.

"I'm not sure I'm allowed. I will have to check with the Choice people and see if it's the clinic they approved or only you."

Unbelievable. They probably billed Choice for the exam too.

The tears made it difficult to see the road as I headed back to my office. I called Choice and inquired. They said anyone who accepted Choice pay would do; I need only let them know in advance who the surgeon would be.

Then I scrolled through doctors who might not only take the Choice program but would also do the surgery in less than five weeks. I found Dr. S. I'd hoped he could and would help me.

After the exam, he said he could do the surgery on the last Tuesday of the month. "But I'm leaving for vacation the next day. I'd hate to leave and then you have some complication." He paused.

In a panic to schedule, I attempted to sell him on the idea. "I'm an excellent coagulator."

He tilted his head. "You could see one of the other doctors should something happen. Not that it ever has, but . . . I'm not comfortable leaving town right after a surgery," he hemmed and hawed.

"I'll be fine. And I have to get this done by the end of the year, or I'll be back trying to get approval for who knows how many months."

He yielded. "Make sure you schedule the follow-up exam for two weeks after the surgery."

My heart sank. "But they said it all had to be done before the end of the year."

"Don't worry about it. The surgery will be done and billed by the end of the month, and the follow-up in January will be included in the price. There won't be additional charges. I'll see you on December 27th."

As I looked around his office, I could see the telltale signs of his Christianity. Not a lot, just pictures and trinkets, but enough to give me confidence in God moving on my behalf.

The doctor even directed me back to the VA for a bacterial infection. "How long has it been going on?" He asked about a strong odor.

"Off and on for a few months?" I said with uncertainty. Had it been longer? "I dismissed it as the death throes of my uterus."

The VA gave me a vaginal suppository, which worked in time for my first date with Dean.

Timing.

A dark cloud loomed over Christmas, with surgery scheduled for two days afterward. But I mustered through and arrived for the excruciatingly early pre-operation preparations. The surgery went well, as did the recovery. At the two-week checkup, he released me for work. I thanked him profusely for taking me with the Choice program. I imagined the pay left a lot to be desired, and he had to commit quickly.

Estrogen Overload

He walked me to the front desk, and I thanked him again, along with the staff. "Because of you, I am free to live my uterus-free life." They assured me they'd never heard it put that way before. (I get that a lot, usually with mouths agape.) I went back to work the next day.

The benefits of the partial hysterectomy were great. It enabled me to unload my purse of an old makeup bag I'd lugged around for years. It contained numerous feminine sanitary products of various strengths or sizes. I ditched the just-in-case towels, and my supply of ibuprofen lasted as it should. The birth control pills went into the trash. My nighttime routine eased a little. During the day, I didn't have the nagging sensation of starting my period or bleeding through again.

A year later, I saw my superstar doctor in the news. Dressed in scrubs, Dr. S. had stopped at four in the morning for gas on the way to deliver a baby at the hospital. A young man had run up to him at the pumps, asking, "My wife is in labor. Can you deliver a baby?" He could. And he did.

Why Didn't I Get a Baseline Test?

Life is good.

Except for all the other things going on in my body.

A lot of this is in retrospect, but I should have had a baseline hormone test done in my twenties or early thirties before things went sideways. As things went haywire, I complained at my annual checkups with the primary care physicians. There were numerous doctors, and the VA rotated me through staff. They tested, but the hormones and thyroid came back normal. Each time.

After the partial hysterectomy, my blood numbers rocked. All the tests were normal. At least normal for a human adult female.

But I wasn't *feeling* normal.

How I wish I could've gone back in time and done a baseline. Then, it would be in my records, and doctors would have something to compare.

If it's not too late, get a hormone test now—right now. Pay for it if you have to.

Without testing when things are good, it's a guessing game with the doctors to get you back to normal. Everyone's different. One doctor told me normal is considered anything between ten and ninety percent with the hormone tests. What if your normal is seventy-eight, but your test result is thirty-two? You are within the normal range, so most doctors won't consider doing something for a normal test result.

But if you show *your* normal is much higher, then your doctor has a happy place to aim for instead of shooting blindly and trying to treat to beat the symptoms. Aimless treatments can take a lot of effort, money, and time to get there.

If only I had done a baseline test.

Should've.

Could've.

Would've.

CHAPTER 3

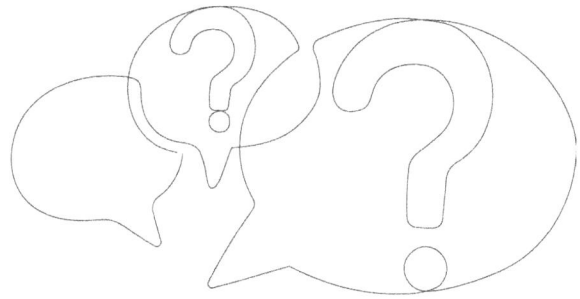

WHAT ARE WE TALKING ABOUT?

Definitions and the Nitty Gritty of Hormones

The three stages of menopause normally start during the mid to late forties or early fifties.

> **The Three Stages of Menopause and Their Symptoms**[1]
>
> 1. Perimenopause
>   - The ovaries produce less and less estrogen during this time, accelerating the decline during the last couple of years. With eggs still being released, even if infrequently, pregnancy can still happen.
>   - Monthly periods get less frequent. When a woman has twelve consecutive months without a period, she is considered menopausal.
>   - Symptoms can include breast tenderness, worsening of premenstrual syndrome (PMS), irregular or skipped periods,

and heavier or lighter periods. Women might also experience racing heart, headaches, joint and muscle aches and pains, a change in sex drive/libido, difficulty concentrating, temporary memory lapses, weight gain, and hair loss/thinning.
2. Menopause
   - During this stage, no eggs are released and estrogen production is greatly reduced.
   - Symptoms can include hot flashes, night sweats and cold flashes, vaginal dryness or discomfort during sex, urinary urgency, insomnia, dry skin, dry eyes, dry mouth. Women can also experience emotional changes, like irritability, mood swings, and mild depression.
3. Postmenopause
   - At this stage, many of the menopause symptoms ease for most women.
   - With the reduction in hormones, women are at a higher risk for heart and bone health conditions.

(The Cleveland Clinic article was careful to mention seeking medical advice to rule out more serious medical concerns if numerous symptoms appear.)

The first stage, called perimenopause, can last almost a decade. This is when the ovaries produce less estrogen, but you still have a period, even if infrequent, and you can nevertheless get pregnant. If it wasn't a party before, premenstrual syndrome (**PMS**) can get worse.

You might have heavier or lighter periods, or they may skip a month, like the worst noncommittal boyfriend you ever had. Almost any horrible thing you can think of can be related to the perimenopausal stage: racing heart, headaches/migraines, weight gain, and hair loss. Other symptoms make you look like an idiot with difficulty

What Are We Talking About?

concentrating and memory lapses. On a regular day, I did well to remember my name.

A woman is considered in the second stage, menopause, when she's gone twelve consecutive months without a period—hard for me to judge without a uterus. I looked to other symptoms to judge my condition, like eggs being released, but it's been a long time since I noticed a twitch from my ovaries. Instead, insomnia and hot flashes riddled my otherwise pleasant constitution. Having been chaste for over two decades, I didn't notice any changes in my sex drive, vaginal dryness, or discomfort during sex. Until I married Dean. On the honeymoon. Good times.

Inadvertently, I attributed the irritability and mood swings to living in a multigenerational home.

Women are considered in the final stage, postmenopause, when all the nonsense stops. But it doesn't mean the party ceases. For some, it's just the beginning. As the hormones plummet, our risk for heart disease and bone health conditions increases.

You might feel like you are going crazy. You might be, or your changing hormone levels might be to blame. Some doctors suggest the worse your PMS was through your reproductive years, the worse menopause might be. There's no proof of this, but doctors still stand firm on this. For me, it has been true.

When hormones decrease, doctors usually recommend hormone replacement therapy (HRT) or bioidentical hormone replacement therapy (BHRT) to help with symptoms. The hormones involved are usually estrogen, progesterone, and testosterone. Estrogen (a group of hormones—estradiol, estriol, and estrone) helps with hot flashes and night sweats, skin and vaginal dryness, as well as sleep, sex drive, and mood. Estradiol, in particular, is known to help with bone health and brain function.[2]

The progesterone your body once made helped regulate your estrogen levels. Some doctors won't prescribe progesterone if you've had your uterus removed, but others are recommending **BHRT** progesterone to help with sleep and cancer prevention. It is also a natural antidepressant, antianxiety, and mood enhancer. Low progesterone is related to brain fog and depression. It helps with sleep and can relieve hot flashes and night sweats.[3]

Testosterone isn't just for men. Women's bodies also produce testosterone, which helps with heart health, libido (sex drive), and muscles. As with the other hormones, there's a crossover of benefits in the areas of sleep, bone density, and brain health.[4]

Experts also suggest dietary changes to include three meals daily, each with protein. Increase your Omega-3 fatty acids through fish, flax seeds, and walnuts. Eliminate refined carbohydrates: sugar (cane, honey, syrup, etc.), white flour (made from modern wheat), and wine. This will help your body burn stored fats and stabilize blood sugar and insulin. Pay attention to the glycemic indexes of foods in your diet.[5] Also, diminish caffeine consumption and quit smoking to reduce hot flashes during perimenopause and menopause.[6]

Or keep the bad diet and vices and enjoy the wild ride.

Sounds like a good time to rethink your choice of Chinese takeout restaurants as well as your diet overall. The more natural, the better. Numerous times lately, I've heard about shopping in the outer sections of the grocery store and staying away from the inside aisles. I have a hard time keeping up with scientific reports like eggs are bad for you, then eggs are good for you, and other changing opinions in the medical community, but it seems nobody is negative toward food you can grow in your backyard. This might be a good time to try a raised garden of your own.

The consensus is for women to see their doctor for guidance first. Then, under your doctor's care, try changing your diet and exercise before you introduce any medication. While I've tried most things known to modern science, I still think it's best to go natural

What Are We Talking About?

when you can. Just because it didn't work for me doesn't mean it won't work for you. We're all different.

The following chapters expound on my experiences with The Change and any remedy I've tried or heard works. Though my body has found little alleviation from symptoms, I'm hoping you or your loved one can find some relief from what can sometimes interfere with daily life. If knowledge is power and an ounce of prevention is worth a pound of cure, then maybe, like me, you will find some consolation in simply putting a name to the pain and knowing this, too, shall pass.

CHAPTER 4

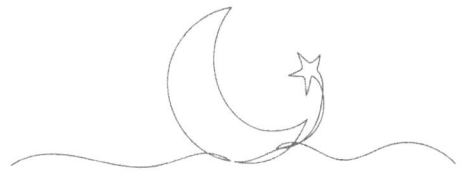

INSOMNIA

An acute case of insomnia developed in 2008 after I turned forty. Sleep is easy until it's not. I'd woken for two or three hours in the middle of the night, but those occurrences only happened once every few weeks. Over the next four years, it morphed into chronic insomnia, with me waking numerous times each night. Instead of staying awake, I could usually go right back to sleep, but when the alarm went off, it felt like I hadn't slept at all. Every night proved to be a challenge, a test I had to pass accompanied by anxiety and pressure.

For random nights with long periods awake or the occasional hard time falling asleep, I built a DVR collection around television shows or movies I'd seen a thousand times and would watch them to fall back asleep. Nothing too interesting because I didn't want to get the blood pumping. However, most nights, my eyes were shut almost 100 percent of the time; nevertheless, every morning, I woke exhausted.

From over-the-counter (OTC) products to numerous items at the health food store, if it worked for the person recommending it or someone they knew, I tried it. Anything legal. I wasn't desperate enough to cruise a particular part of town for illicit drugs. Not at that point.

In 2012, at forty-five, I complained at my monthly scrapbooking meetings. All the older (than me) ladies swore it must be hormones. All of them.

"It's The Change. I didn't sleep for years until I came out on the other side," one lady said.

Another said, "I still sweat through my pajamas a couple of times per week."

They all piled on, and I should've listened, but I didn't. And neither did the VA, who told me that same year my hormone test results landed in the normal range, so not to worry.

My primary care physician at the VA ran tests to rule out anything benign or malignant. Then he did more tests. As the results came back normal, he moved on to the next test. During this time, he also referred me to a sleep hygiene class.

Sleep Hygiene Class

Of the ten sufferers in the group class, only I had sleep maintenance insomnia. The others all had sleep onset insomnia—they all complained of not falling asleep quickly or waking for hours in the middle of the night. And the only one not on 100 percent disability or retired military and sitting happily on a full pension? Yep, me. Nope, I alone struggled to get to an eight-to-five job. And I was the only one under sixty years old.

We hung in there week by week as Dr. C. guided us through stacks of handouts from *Cognitive Behavioral Treatment of Insomnia*.[1]

Week 1—Sleep Education and Stimulus Control. I scored a seventeen on the self-evaluation test, which earned me a moderate severity rating in the Chronic Insomnia category.[2] The clinical

Insomnia

psychologist then educated us on sleep cycles and stimulus control. She educated us on the benefits of waking at a regular time, even on the weekends. (What? No catching up?) After calming the class down, she then extolled the advantages of using the bed only for sleep (and sex, but no problem there) and sleeping only in your bed, not the recliner or couch.

Again, Dr. C. had to tell us to simmer down. The next point of only going to bed when you're tired seemed to conflict with setting a schedule, but she added we were not to stay in bed while awake for more than fifteen minutes. "Get up and read in a chair or some other calm activity, nothing stimulating, like physical exercise, smoking, or television. Practice breathing correctly or journal, but don't go back to bed until you're sleepy."

I failed to do any of it the right way.

The facilitator went over some of the causes of insomnia, like sleep apnea, where you stop breathing numerous times per minute throughout the night. The instructor covered some of the things we could do on our own to help alleviate insomnia, like deep breathing exercises, diet, and physical activities to reduce anxiety and depression.

 Tip: Avoid screen time within an hour of bedtime, and don't watch anything in the middle of the night. The blue light from computers, smartphones, tablets, and televisions suppresses melatonin in the brain and triggers sleeplessness. If you simply must, try blue light filtering glasses.

Finally, she pressed, "No napping during the day." The room erupted in disapproval. I'd never been a good napper and had no problem following that particular rule. As an adult, the naps I'd taken could be counted on one hand—a little too highly strung to relax enough to drift off during the day; the feeling of missing out on something good always got the better of me.

Insomnia is not like the occasional bad night of sleep, where you can make up for the interrupted sleep. Naps exacerbate the problem and compound the issue.

Week 2—Sleep Restriction, Sleep Efficiency, and Sleep Hygiene. Dr. C. explained sleep efficiency (SE), which is the total sleep time divided by the total time in bed. You end up with a percentage: 85 percent for adults under sixty-five years old, and 80 percent for adults over sixty-five is the goal. They'd skewed the test toward those whose eyes were wide open during the night, unlike me. (Example: If John is in bed from 11:00 p.m. until 7:00 a.m., then his total time in bed is eight hours. If he is awake from 1:00 a.m. until 4:00 a.m., then his total sleep time is five hours. His SE is five divided by eight, or 62.5 percent.) The total time asleep remained elusive for my type of insomnia, especially without the wrist devices so many of us now have, which track your sleep for you.

She then reviewed the sleep hygiene instructions.

Sleep Hygiene Instructions[3]

- Restrict your time in bed to help get deeper sleep and stay asleep.
- Get up at the same time each day, even on the weekends.
- Exercise regularly, but not within one hour of bedtime.[4]
- Make your bedroom comfortable, free of noise and light, and at the right temperature—not too hot or too cold.
- Eat regular meals, but don't go to bed with a belly full of greasy or heavy foods. Eat a snack before bed, if needed, so hunger doesn't interrupt sleep.
- Cut down on liquids in the last three hours before bedtime.
- Eliminate caffeine products.
- Avoid alcohol, which can cause awakenings during the night.

- Avoid nicotine, especially before bedtime.
- Work on your problems and planning activities well before bedtime. Write them down to get them out of your head. Worry can interrupt sleep or cause shallow sleep.
- Don't struggle to get to sleep. The frustration can be problematic. Leave the bed and do a nonstimulating activity, like reading. Return to bed only when sleepy.
- Cover or remove the clock to avoid clock-watching frustrations.
- Avoid naps.

Week 3—Cognitive Therapy. The facilitator had us fill out a questionnaire and consider negative thoughts that might interfere with sleep. What do you think about when you wake up? Do you think about the sleep issue and its negative impact on your life, such as your health or job? What is the estimated probability of negative consequences? She made us see those fearful thoughts during the night that probably would never happen. Then she told us to come up with a positive thought to replace the negative thought and to say it over and over out loud.

Little Susan from *Miracle on 34th Street* came to mind, slumped on the car's bench seat, repeating, "I believe, I believe. It's silly, but I believe."

We then evaluated our belief system about sleep. The form had numerous statements to help control anxiety and irrational thoughts.

Finally, the psychologist gave us a list of things to do to promote good sleep hygiene.

Promote Sleep Hygiene

In the Evening, Before Bedtime—Nothing Too Exciting
- Pick out clothes for the morning
- Make a lunch for work

- Take a bath or long shower
- Listen to relaxing or instrumental music
- Shred documents
- Watch a mundane television show
- Polish your shoes
- Iron or mend clothing
- Stretch to relax muscles
- Do your nails
- Knit or other crafts

During the Night—Bore Yourself Back to Sleep
- Peruse a catalog
- Sort through bills (but don't pay them, it could get you too worked up!)
- Play solitaire online or with cards
- Read a book
- Call a friend in another time zone (know any missionaries in China?)
- Clean out the refrigerator
- Make a grocery shopping list (to fill your now empty fridge)

    She told us to create a snooze-fest of activities—a list of boring activities to lull us back to sleep. Since my heavy eyes close quickly after each awakening, I found the nighttime list useless. Also, I'm not a straight-A student, but I noticed an inconsistency within the lists and her teachings during the first week. When I pointed out the blue-light screen activity on her list of before-bedtime activities, she glared at me as if I wore the troublemaker hat. Surely that label belonged to Mike, the part-time real estate agent, not I, ma'am!

    My snarky attitude probably contributed to me not staying past my initial four-year enlistment in the army. Besides, they always stripped the fun out of everything.

Insomnia

Week 4—Relaxation Training and Relapse Prevention. The doctor went over easy relaxation techniques. It reminded me of another group-counseling class the military made me do for irritable bowel syndrome (IBS), where they pretty much told me I had to be someone else—not my usual uptight type A personality.

"Everyone can learn to relax." She then further expounded, "At least one of these techniques will work for you."

Half of the suggested methods harkened to the new age mumbo jumbo the Baptist church warned me about and, later, saw people delivered from in other churches. I settled on deep breathing. By taking a deep breath and slowly releasing it—take twice as long to exhale as inhale—it's supposed to ease you back into sleep. In the instances when I couldn't just roll over and fall quickly back to sleep, I practiced my breathing, releasing calming endorphins. Though deep breathing didn't turn out to be a magic sleep pill, I used it almost weekly, usually in the middle of traffic during my harrowing commute to the office; I still do.

The psychologist then left us with a sleep diary to fill out during the following week before our next session. It had questions like "What time did you get into bed?" and "What time did you try to go to sleep?" It felt like a trick because they'd already told us not to get into bed until we were ready to sleep. The next question asked how long it took to go to sleep. How would you know if you covered or removed your clock? The frustration from this question prompted me to practice my deep breaths.

Week 5—Long-Term Habits and Relapse Prevention. Dr. C. reiterated having constant bedtimes and wake-up times. Each student then explained their plan for how to handle awakenings, and as discussed during the fourth week, I chose deep breaths. We looked over our sleep logs and evaluated our sleep again with the Insomnia Severity Index. My score improved to thirteen, even though sleep had not improved. I could not judge myself accurately because they had designed this class for the other kind of insomniacs. The rest of the session dealt with PTSD and nightmares.

After another year of tests, prescriptions, and continued lack of sleep, my primary care physician sent me an hour down the road to the VA Lake Baldwin facility to do a sleep study to see if they could find a reason.

The Sleep Study

During check-in, the technician asked, "Are you waking from night terrors or night sweats?"

"No."

"Do you have someone complaining you snore?"

In an opportunity to share my stellar streak of abstinence approaching two decades, I explained only my mother would know from our scrapbooking or vacation trips, and she'd never complained to me.

The tech moved on after not calling me a freak of nature or a liar, except with his facial expression. "Do you think you might have restless leg syndrome (RLS)? Are the sheets or blankets all messed up when you wake, or in other words, do you wake up twisted in them?"

"Nope." I didn't share that I'm the type who makes my bed each morning. After I wake, there is such an insignificant change in the bedding, making it again is a snap. I didn't want notes indicating obsessive control in my file, not after the raised eyebrow from the abstinence fact.

"So, what makes you think you might have a sleep issue?"

"Because I feel like the Princess and the Pea—I'm never comfortable for long. It feels like I wake twenty times during the night as if I'm sleeping in the in-between stage. When the alarm goes off in the morning, I'm exhausted, like I'd never slept at all. Occasionally,

Insomnia

I can't go back to sleep for two or three hours in the middle of the night."

The large sleep study room I'd imagined had a king-sized bed, a beige silk bedspread with a small jacquard pattern and shams to match, crisp white sheets folded over the spread, and king-sized comfy pillows. I pictured twin nightstands in a modern box style with table lamps. The beige carpet completed the serene room ambiance.

Instead, he showed me to a private hospital-like room, not at all like the upscale spa hotel room I'd envisioned. No double, queen, or king bed as I imagined, just a single-wide hospital bed made with crisp white sheets—the only thing I'd guessed right. They spent the next hour hooking me up to a plethora of cables and cords from head to foot. I particularly remember the plaster leads they used on my scalp to adhere the cranial lines and skull cap. They grouped the wires with a band, then attached the wad to my arm and extended the cluster to a portable machine to record my vitals and other signals.

Channel surfing on TV occupied my time while they connected the wires to the other patients during the eight o'clock hour. (The irony of having a television with its forbidden blue light in the sleep study room was not lost on me.) Worried I wouldn't get any sleep with the wired skull cap, I surprisingly drifted off right after they announced lights out at nine. Around three a.m. I pushed a button to help me get out of bed to use the bathroom. At five-thirty, they woke me to go home. Thankful for what seemed like a typical lousy night's sleep, I hadn't wasted my time or theirs. Similar to any other medical test technician, they gave me no answers. "The doctor will go over the test results with you."

A couple of weeks later, my primary care physician explained how the test showed no signs of sleep apnea or restless leg syndrome, the two main issues found in a sleep test. "You had thirty-three arousals, and the test shows you only got about 20 percent each of the REM and the deep restorative sleep you need."

"So, it's exactly what I thought happened."

"It would seem so, but there were alpha wave intrusions, too, which are indicators of pain." He poked and prodded my body, then noted, "You have eleven of the nineteen pain sensitivity points for fibromyalgia."

"I don't think it's fibromyalgia. I know someone with that, and it's just a cluster of symptoms, not a disease, right?"

"Yes, but like other conditions, there can be degrees," he said.

I replied, "I think I'm only sore because I'm tossing and turning all night."

Ignoring me, he prescribed venlafaxine for the fibromyalgia, which I didn't have. After four months, he agreed with me but stepped me down too quickly. He took me off the drug by reducing the medication only once instead of the three or four increments recommended by the multitude of opinions on the internet. My head spun, and it reminded me of the dizziness you feel when a crystal is loose in the inner ear.

One day, while exiting a highway on the east side of Orlando on my way back from yet another VA doctor appointment, I stopped at the end of the exit ramp. I glanced left to check for a break in traffic to merge onto another highway—all clear. Suddenly, my head vibrated like a tuning fork struck hard on a solid surface.

For the rest of the drive, with my eyes forward, I didn't turn my head for anything to avoid dizziness. I made sure to stay in the right-hand lane and to turn only when necessary. After getting home, I vowed to drive only when necessary, which included that evening's chiropractor appointment. Suspecting a loose crystal in my ear, he attempted to get it back in place using the Epley maneuver. It's like the little, wooden cube game you tilt to get the metal balls into the holes. After two attempts with no positive results, I drove home, avoiding the side and rearview mirrors. Eyes forward.

Once home, I searched the web and found the culprit: venlafaxine—another drug for sleep that didn't work and only gave me bad side effects. Some people online complained their heads spun for up to two months. I only had it for a mere two weeks. With my hand inches from my face as my focal point, I moved around and used my peripheral vision. When I used that method, I kept the spinning to a minimum.

They don't call it "practicing medicine" for nothing. After three long years of horrible sleep, my primary care physician finally referred me to a sleep specialist.

The Sleep Specialist

The specialist reiterated that I didn't have regular insomnia with long periods of being wide awake, the kind where you could do something productive, like clean the house or write a book. I had the kind where I failed to stay asleep. I had numerous arousals but fell back to sleep quickly and didn't get the deeper levels of sleep—REM and deep restorative sleep. I shut my eyes for 95 percent of the night but awoke exhausted each morning.

He asked me to explain how the lack of sleep affected me.

I used to be graceful. I told him I'd taken gymnastics and ballet classes as a child and teenager. However, due to a lack of quality sleep, I ran into walls, doors, and corners of desks and almost missed my work chair at least once a week. For the first time in my life, I lacked coordination. I'd broken numerous glasses and dishes—more than all the previous years combined.

In my family, my sister earned the title of Crash Kim. They called me Safety Sal, but no more. I'd driven the past years with my car sporting a protective cover across the grill to cover the hole in the front bumper caused by a work truck's tow ball when the driver stopped short in front of me—a scenario I should've seen coming. I've also started rubbing curbs with my tires regularly.

For the past several years, since my mid-forties, I've walked around exhausted all the time. Every nook beckoned me to lie down to take a nap, except I usually couldn't sleep unless I had a fever. I'm the high-strung type of personality, which made it hard to settle in for a quick nap. Normally, there had to be at least a three-hour window with nothing on the schedule before I could relax enough to drift off.

The last time I'd successfully napped without a fever was thirty years ago, during my army years. I'd set my alarm wrong and missed flag duty. I paid for it with extra duty. It reiterated the feeling of missing out on something if I took a nap. Not that I'm supposed to nap with insomnia anyhow.

My concentration and awareness have also suffered. I often lose my train of thought mid-sentence and have developed the horrible habit of interrupting others' conversations to add my two cents before the thought escapes me. I've driven blocks without recalling the distance traveled.

With raw nerves, my patience ran short. Seemingly, everything I put my hands to went awry. (As I've told my husband, Dean, a hundred times already, "It's so hard being me.") Even the easiest tasks became more difficult, and emotions ran high.

For the better part of two years, the sleep specialist prescribed more than a dozen different medications. I couldn't try some drugs because they'd impair driving in the morning. And I needed to drive to work five days a week to spoil myself with the essentials of life, like food and shelter, which required money . . . entailing work in my case. A vicious circle.

I was hoping for a magic sleeping pill that would produce results no matter what state I was in. I wanted to be able to turn off

Insomnia

my brain like you see in older movies, such as *The Man Who Knew Too Much*, when the wife gets frantic over their missing child. One minute, she's crying and weeping, the next, she's unconscious. Sweet sleep. The magic of Hollywood.

Most of the drugs the expert prescribed were anti-depressants with side effects of drowsiness. I already felt tired all the time and didn't have problems falling asleep, but I tried them nonetheless with no success. Jumping through the government hoops, I tried everything they threw at me that wouldn't make me a zombie the next day.

Finally, I had arrived—something I'd recognized from television commercials: Ambien. I knew others had reported eating or driving without any recollection the next day, but desperate people will try anything. I gulped them down for a couple of weeks with no change.

A year later, another doctor prescribed Ambien as the generic zolpidem. I didn't recognize it as such and fell for it again. I had a conversation with a conference roommate but didn't remember it the next morning. I had a friend who'd also taken Ambien for sleep. They institutionalized him for three days for self-harm potential while they figured out the brand-new psychiatric problem that he'd never experienced before.

Ambien.

Turns out it's a drug they usually reserve for end-of-life patients with nothing to lose. It didn't help me sleep any better. It only made me not remember sleeping horribly. Not a cure, only a bandage. The upside is that not being aware of the bad slumber can help keep you from freaking out about it; avoiding the stress of rousing can help you fall back asleep more quickly.

Alas, none of the medications I tried gave me additional or deeper sleep. I only achieved the usual four broken hours I could get without assistance.

VA nurses called to ensure I handled each prescription well enough. They also verified that I didn't get screen time too late and that my reading materials didn't excite me.

I got none of the benefits but often felt the side effects. Nothing as bad as the head-spinning vertigo from venlafaxine, but frustrating nonetheless.

After depleting his medication list, the specialist cut me loose. "We've tried everything. There's nothing else I can give you."

"How about Michael Jackson's anesthesiologist's phone number? I'm just kidding. But seriously, do you have the number?" We both got a good laugh. (I come from a long line of laugh-or-cry people; we choose to laugh . . . usually.)

"I would, but I don't have it, and that kind of sleep is the high-level sleep like you're getting now."

Too bad. But it did save me from dumpster diving behind the hospitals looking for partially spent canisters of general anesthesia gas.

The Christian Mental Health Counselor

With the psych-wing visit coming as the next step at the VA, I tried heading it off at the pass. I made an appointment with a local Christian mental health counselor. I explained my difficulties and what I'd already tried on my own and through the VA.

Shelly said, "It could be hormones, but I think you have a couple of other things affecting you too. You seem stuck in a job that doesn't get you out of bed in the morning. I can give you some job-hunting tips, but you'll have to do it on your own. The other item is what you feel is an unanswered promise from the Lord for a husband."

Yes, she understood me. "I do feel stuck . . . in both of them."

She gave me some suggestions on searching for a new job. I did find a couple of jobs, but they were out of the area. Besides, it's a catch-22. How do you start a new job if you can't guarantee you'll be there at 8:00 a.m. each day for a ninety-day probationary period, let alone long-term? Double stuck. At least my current boss understood with the occasional late mornings and numerous appointments as long as the work got done, which it did.

"About the husband?" I asked.

"Enlarge your circles. I want you to hear me." Shelly leaned forward in her chair toward me. "Please hear me. I'm not saying to leave your current church. I want you to find a Bible study at a larger church."

My heart sank. "Do you mean a singles group? I don't think I can go through it again, twenty years older now."

"Not necessarily. A women's group will have ladies with brothers, cousins, uncles, and nephews. You need to meet more people."

Heeding her advice, I followed some friends down the road to a larger church. Within the first month, I met a man, and we eventually married. It didn't improve my sleep, but I loved seeing God move and fulfill a promise decades in the making. In the meantime . . .

The Psychiatrist

After the sleep doctor, while still seeing Shelly, I acquiesced and went over to the psych wing of the VA in Viera. I'd previously dragged my feet because I'd heard horror stories in the news about vets losing their concealed carry permits for guns.

In the spring of 2016, a Brevard County detective on behalf of the FBI informed me that ISIS had put me on one of their kill lists. I'd had my permit for years but never took advantage of it until then. Immediately, I started carrying for protection, not as much for me as for loved ones. I didn't want to risk losing my permit because of anything a shrink might say.

A nurse called to make the appointment, and I expressed my concerns. She assured me those were extreme cases of mental illness and PTSD, where lives were truly at risk. She then reassured me I would not lose my permit simply for seeing a psychiatrist.

First, as part of the process, they sent me to a psychologist. After chatting with him, he decided I might benefit from the "good drugs" on the psychiatric wing but said he had to try a couple of other drugs first. Those trials took over a month each. In the meantime, he sent over the referral. Another month passed before the appointment with a psychiatrist.

When I eventually sat across from her desk, she asked what medications I'd already tried.

"I can't pronounce most of them, let alone remember anything these days. Don't you have the list of meds in my records?"

"It's a different system in Orlando."

She clicked around on her desktop computer for another few minutes while she asked questions.

My answers were honest. I wanted drugs. I wanted to sleep.

Then it happened . . .

"Have you tried"—she swiveled in her chair from the computer to face me—"melatonin?"

My head swam in the possibilities of the question's reality. I glanced around the office, looking for a hidden camera, Ashton Kutcher, and his Punked show. I wondered if she was messing with me to get a certain response.

No, she sat seriously and waited for my reply to her question about me trying an OTC item found at numerous grocery and health food stores.

Had I braved the arduous journey of getting to this particular doctor to hear the doctor recommend a drugstore item? I wanted to come over the desk and cause bodily harm, but I miraculously maintained my composure, trying not to let the rising anger get the best of me. I pursed my lips and parsed each word to make sure I didn't end up leaving in a straitjacket or handcuffs. "Yes. In the past five years, out of sheer exhaustion and desperation, I have tried melatonin in varying strengths at different times."

"Have you tried it with your current medication?"

She got me there. "No, I have not." I couldn't lie. I wouldn't lie. What if this oversimplified suggestion held the answer?

"I've gotten great results adding melatonin to my own medication."

Her medication? Which one? Unbelievably, she'd prescribed something because it worked for her. I doubted her professionalism. Did she not have access to a Physicians' Desk Reference?

"I want you to keep taking what the psychologist prescribed and add the melatonin to it for six weeks. You can pick it up at the window on your way out. And they'll call you for a follow-up appointment in eight weeks."

If it weren't the answer, it would cost me another two months of sleep. Every delay ate away at my fortitude, not to mention another eleven dollars in copay. It had been cheaper just buying it at a local store—a double whammy.

2017—new year, new me. Not quite. The psychiatrist also referred me to Orlando's Lake Baldwin VA facility for attention deficit disorder and attention-deficit/hyperactivity disorder (ADD/ADHD) testing.

At least the Orlando appointment took place after work, and I didn't have to use my yearly allocated vacation time to drive to the VA hospital. Small mercies. I told the doctor right away what I thought about the referral for testing. "I have no idea what one has to do with the other, and I'm sorry the psychiatrist is wasting both of our time."

He let me go on for a bit.

"How can I have ADD/ADHD if caffeine jacks me?"

Hot Mess Express

He showed great patience and reminded me to be completely honest with my answers. Afterward, he went over the test results, telling me I didn't have anything close to an ADD/ADHD diagnosis. "You do have issues, but nothing medicine would help."

He wasn't wrong. I know I have issues; don't we all? But of this particular kind, several teachers had already made me keenly aware. My mother had received a call from my elementary teacher with great concern over my not remembering a quiz that day. I'm sure there were numerous notes on report cards too. Some didn't bother to notify my parents.

As before, the melatonin did nothing for my sleep, and I showed back up for the psychiatrist after two months, in late February . . . holding my tongue.

"How about topiramate? Have you tried it? It's an anti-seizure medication. I tried it once. Took it when I left work and then got lost by the time I got to my street, and I'd lived there for over seven years."

A smile adorned my face, but on the inside, I wanted to punch her. I didn't care for her form of doctoring, shirking the panel studies for her own experiences with the drugs. How is this woman practicing medicine anywhere? "Sure, let's try it."

On the way home with the drug, I called my friend with seizure experiences. She said she tolerated the brand-name version of the drug but not the generic form prescribed for me. "Watch out for the buzzing."

"What buzzing?"

She hesitated and then said, "It's like a bunch of bees buzzing in your head." Then she quickly added, "But that's just me. Maybe you won't experience it."

Insomnia

If only.

During the night, my head buzzed exactly as she'd described it. Not only did I not sleep any better, but I didn't think I'd slept at all, like in a constant state of awareness, even with my eyes closed.

Anger set in as I tossed and turned.

A rage rose inside me, like when she offered melatonin. I went to work dead on my feet. When I got the chance, I called to cancel my next appointment with her. They asked why, and I told them, holding nothing back.

"You can come in and fill out some paperwork requesting a new doctor."

With additional vacation time wasted, I made the half-hour trek back down to the Viera VA clinic and filled out the paperwork.

> **Over-the-Counter Solutions for Sleep**[5]
>
> **Melatonin**—Your brain makes this naturally and builds to the highest levels in the evening, promoting sleep.
>
> **Valerian**—Sounds more like a movie title than a plant, but this root treats anxiety and promotes sleep and insomnia.
>
> **Chamomile**—I used it as a tea and with lavender as a scented bubble bath. Chamomile is known as an anti-inflammatory and antibacterial with a calming effect.
>
> **Tryptophan**—It makes millions drowsy every Thanksgiving, especially for those who eat a turkey dinner and then sit on a recliner. Also present in milk—I've tried it straight from the fridge or warmed at bedtime.

Someone took it from me and said I'd get a call to schedule with a new psychiatrist.

The call never came, and I didn't reach out for another appointment. By then, I determined hormones were to blame.

The OTC generic sleep aid with diphenhydramine, which is the active ingredient in Tylenol PM or ZzzQuil, kept me from tossing too much—more likely, it made me not remember all the tossing and turning. According to the Fitbit my mother gave to me as a birthday gift the previous year, it reported the same as the sleep study: numerous awakenings and few segments of actual sleep.

The Health Food Store

Through my search to return to restful sleep, I frequently visited the health food store. Perhaps I am very different than the average person, but I couldn't find anything helpful.

My sister is a forensic scientist and reads scientific journals and studies for fun, if you can imagine. She swears the natural remedies found at the local store or online are all rubbish. "If there is any relief, then it's a placebo effect."

My reply to her was, "I'd kill for a placebo effect right about now."

The friendly people of the local health food store suggested melatonin, valerian, and chamomile. Tryptophan is also known to knock out quite a few after their Thanksgiving Day turkey dinner. I'd tried it in supplement form too.

I tried everything people recommended if it worked for either them or someone they personally knew. But I kept coming back to the diphenhydramine. It's bad enough to struggle through the night, but if you're aware of waking and have no memories of the battle, then all the better.

Word on the street is that redheads are a bit medicine-resistant. Again, my sister says it's malarkey, but it would explain why I never got relief from OTC or the meds prescribed to me.

The Many Side Effects of Insomnia

Insomnia makes many tasks more difficult. Driving is a doozy. I have no patience for slow or crazy drivers, even if I am one. Like

Insomnia

a barn-bound trail horse, I have to drive with a map app on my phone if I want to go anywhere other than home or work. Too often, I didn't realize I'd missed my intended stop until I pulled into my driveway. I've hit more curbs in the past five years than in the previous thirty-five.

Cruise control is my new best friend. I use it to avoid going too fast or too slow. I have zero concentration and have never prayed more for traveling mercies. I have never nodded off but occasionally can't recall driving the previous two miles. Experts equate it to a hypnotic trance. Everybody experiences this from time to time, but it's almost daily for me.

The decline in our societal manners is clearly demonstrated on our roads. With a lack of courtesy, my commute became more like driving a gauntlet (see the Clint Eastwood movie *The Gauntlet* or the remake with Bruce Willis, *16 Blocks*). People have forgotten that using blinkers serves more than simply courtesy because it's the law—you can get a ticket for an illegal lane change for not using them. Most drivers seem unwilling to make a U-turn. They'd rather risk your life with theirs to cross three lanes of traffic to avoid missing their turn (all done without a blinker, of course).

If the posted speed limit is forty-five, the average person is going closer to fifty-five. Yet we also have an abundance of "snowbirds"—retirees who come down to Florida from the northeast for the winter. They arrive in October and stay until the snow stops in their home state. With the additional cars on the roads, it takes longer to get anywhere. Many snowbirds use an abundance of caution while driving, often going under the speed limit.

With the combination of aggressive drivers and overly cautious ones, operating a motor vehicle starts to resemble a video game—not the benign Mario Kart or Frogger type, but more like Grand Theft Auto, where you get extra points for sordid jobs. We have a caution zone along my route, which gets interesting as the two types of drivers intersect. According to the county and state traffic engineers, the flashing lights surrounding the yellow 35 MPH sign do not indicate a school zone. Since US1 runs along the side of the school and the front of the school is on a side street, it is only cautionary. I'd only seen five children in three years in the caged crossover, which emptied into a fenced schoolyard. Yes, I counted out of frustration and in preparation for any court action against me one day in the future.

A Florida Department of Transportation engineer compared it to an interstate exit with a sharp curve. I stated that few people are aware of this, and most people are slow to under forty miles per hour while others push sixty or more, creating the perfect setup for an accident or road rage scenario. I expounded on how shocked I am each day when I make it through their caution zone in one piece. I asked him to reconsider the signage, threatening to stand out there with posters informing other drivers that the speed limit is fifty-five and they won't get a speeding ticket.

He said he'd reconsider.

Many moons later, the zone remains. I might look into renting a gas-powered digital sign to educate my fellow travelers. In the meantime, that aspect of my morning drive (more like a mourning drive) keeps my blood flowing and adrenaline pumping to get me to my office at the other end of the county. I'm so busy white-knuckling the steering wheel that I arrive with most of my coffee left in the travel mug.

My day job is also more difficult. Each year at the office, I'm surprised when I receive a bonus instead of a layoff notice. My exceedingly understanding boss said, "I don't keep you here because you're perfect. I keep you around because I can trust you not to run off with the money."

Reassuring since I'm the bookkeeper.

He'd have every right to fire me. Several times per month, I called in to say I'd be late due to another bad night of sleep. I'm

Insomnia

not saying the other nights are good, but sometimes I can't function on three to four hours of broken sleep. I'm normally in well before noon and make up the time when necessary, but I am far from perfect. Once, I forgot to enter a bill to pay and didn't realize until the VISA representative called. A couple of weeks ago, I had one of those conversations and then realized another blunder on the same day. These types of mistakes don't usually cost us anything, but they can't be confidence-builders for the boss.

Concentration on any task makes everything more challenging. In full disclosure, I've always struggled in the pay-attention and remember-anything departments. Combine it with reduced faculties due to insomnia, and that's where things get fun.

In a previous home, I had a record three times for going back upstairs in the two-story townhouse because I'd forgotten something.

Went upstairs to get the item.

Forgot when I reached the top.

I went back down and then remembered when I reached the ground floor.

Three times!

I purposed never again to own a house with multiple levels.

Now I forget in less than ten footsteps. My brother has a saying that Dean and I have adopted: "since-yuhs." I think he adapted it from Jeff Foxworthy. Since-yuhs means *since you are going to* [fill in the blank], *will you get me a* [fill in the blank]?

Dean uses this all the time, at least in principle, if not in the exact phrase. "Are you going to the kitchen? I'm calling since-yuhs. Bring me a bottle of water? Thanks!" (Don't get your feminist panties in a twist, I use it on him just as much.)

Because I can barely remember my name, my execution of such tasks often fails. I bring my plate into the kitchen, rinse it, load the dishwasher, and put away the tray. However, before I can get the water from the fridge, I empty the drain rack, pick up a stray crumb, and use the bathroom.

The next thing I know, I'm sitting on the couch with Dean looking at me. "Really?"

Then I remembered what I'd forgotten. I have even pulled that same stunt two or three times in a row. A smarter person would get the water first, then return to piddle around the kitchen. But I, on the other hand, love to let all my messiness hang out for everyone to see.

Occasionally, I've caught myself "sleeping" with my eyes open. In reality, it's deep thinking without blinking. I have an army yearbook from basic training with a picture of me during sheer exhaustion. The old-timers call it the thousand-yard stare, but with me, it's not wartime with an enemy in the distance.

Both Dean and my brother are big-time nappers. They enjoy naps and are good at them. On the other hand, I'm a notoriously bad napper. As I mentioned before, unless I have a fever, it's not happening. The whole thing is bizarre—I walk around exhausted, spying every nook and cranny in any building as a good spot to get some shut-eye. Yet I fail when I try to nap in a comfortable, safe space at home (not in public).

When Dean and I dated, he suggested I try to take a nap. Later in the day, I told him, "I tried, but after forty minutes, I couldn't. I pulled the ripcord and gave up."

He said, "I don't understand. How does someone fail at napping?"

Indeed. Yet I'm proof after a lifetime of failed siestas.

My brother, Joe, said, "Just lay down and close your eyes." He stops short of saying, "Duh!"

If only.

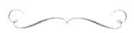

Insomnia

In my early fifties, ten years into the sleep issue, I begged for drugs again. The VA sent me to another psychologist before any psychiatrist capable of writing prescriptions for the good stuff. I'd previously rejected any drug that would've given me a DUI on my daily commute or kept me in a residual brain fog until lunchtime because of my bookkeeping job.

The psychologist met with me online and suggested two apps. The first app helped with mindfulness to keep me from stressing out. I liked the deep breathing exercise, but the others heralded notes of mysticism. Pass. The second app logged my sleep. I felt it only replicated what my Fitbit already did. Nonetheless, I duplicated the info for a week before the surprise. On the seventh day of logging my nighttime activities, the app recommended a new bedtime. Sleep restriction.

I'd refused to try it during the first or second year because I didn't have the luxury of being dead to the world for two months. It turns out that the process can take up to four months to retrain the body and sleep well while in bed. But after a decade of terrible slumber, I relented. I kept in mind I could always quit and go back to my normal wretchedness. The app made me pick a wake time—one time for each of the seven days. I bid farewell to sleep-in Saturdays and hello to 6:15 a.m.

The wake time remained the same throughout the process, and my sleep window shortened over the next four weeks to 12:45 a.m. Surprisingly, I felt no more misery than before the sleep restriction, but staying awake until the prescribed bedtime proved a challenge. The app reminded me to maintain good sleep hygiene: do nothing in bed except sleep (or sex), get out of bed if awake for fifteen-plus minutes, and no tech-screen blue light before crawling in. So, I came up with a list of quiet activities to entertain myself after Dean went to bed each night.

Puzzles worked until they didn't. One time, I caught myself dozing for a moment with my arm in the air, puzzle piece in hand, mid-placement. Crafts helped for a few nights as I added gold fabric paint to my new sea turtle bed shams. When that project ended, I thought about starting on the corresponding comforter but had mercy on Dean; better to let him adjust little by little to the girly embellishments.

Finally, I discovered a true crime miniseries about a surgeon in Texas who had other surgeons wondering if he maimed and killed on purpose or because of his ineptitude. Careful of the TV and tech screens' blue light, which suppresses the brain's natural melatonin and triggers sleeplessness, I wore blue light filtering glasses within two hours of bedtime. I turned down the volume and turned on the closed captioning so as not to wake Dean.

As each activity began to fail for the night, I moved on to another, eventually ending up with a book for the final fifteen to thirty minutes. The routine eventually helped to solidify my ability to stay awake until bedtime and stay asleep until wake time, or at least mostly. Even though my sleep ratio (time asleep divided by total time in bed) averaged just over 90 percent, which is the minimal goal, the app continued to suggest a quarter to one. I contacted my psychologist.

In desperation, I told her, "I need light at the end of the tunnel."

She advised me to add fifteen to twenty minutes weekly when I scored 90 percent or more. Naturally, I added a maximum of twenty minutes each week to the time in bed, allowing myself to go to bed earlier and earlier.

After two months, I finally got to meet with the psychologist for the drugs. I'd begged for anyone but the doctor they'd previously set me up with. So, they gave me one with a former Soviet Union/Russian accent. Surreal, as the Ukrainian war mounted in the news. As Dr. M. navigated his Ws while rolling his Rs, he cracked open my brain with a series of questions. I thought I'd merely answered his kuh-vestions, but he pulled at threads and started weaving a tapestry filled with ADD/ADHD and various mental health disorders.

Insomnia

Nope, nada, nyet. Sorry, better luck next time. I liked him, but after a fun-filled hour-long cranial probe, I didn't care to be under his microscope again.

He explained that sleep restriction and drugs both worked for insomnia, but it's an either/or situation. He further divulged that he'd have tried the same drugs the sleep specialist gave me at first onset. Since they didn't work then, he wouldn't prescribe them now. We both agreed that with my recent progress in sleep, I'd maintain the current course. I explained to him that I'd only requested any drugs for sleep as a stopgap until my appointment the next month at a clinic specializing in hormones.

After some setbacks, I got stuck at a bedtime of 10:30 p.m. for about six weeks. I quit the stringent schedule and allowed for a later wake time when possible, but I mostly kept the bedtime, with my brain still waking close to the regimented wake time anyway. I kept plugging in the Fitbit's report as the app finally eased on my bedtime—not that it mattered by then.

Since Dr. M. killed any expectation of a magic sleeping pill existing, I eagerly clung to the possibilities the hormone clinic held for me, even if it meant paying cash out of pocket.

After several recommendations, I settled on a local clinic specializing in hormones for both men and women. Those recommending the clinic said they'd received relief after only three months. I gave it a year with zero improvements. I finally told them I could be miserable for free at the VA.

With my tail tucked between my legs, I made another appointment at the VA with a gynecologist. Defeated and with both hands up, I told her I'd surrendered. The doctor suggested we back down on the estradiol patch to the lower dose and continue with the progesterone pills each night. My testosterone levels were always at a decent level, so we didn't mess with it.

Hot Mess Express

Dr. O. briefly went over the benefits of estradiol and progesterone and sent me on my way. I already knew the health benefits from dealing with the hormone clinic. I shuffled out with pretty much the same prescriptions, the same symptoms, and my original mantra, "This too shall pass. This too shall pass."

Months later, I'd forgotten to take my progesterone one night. Not wanting to miss a whole day, I took it the next morning when I found it at the foot of the bed where I'd knocked it the night before when turning down the bed comforter. Within an hour I felt drunk (at 10 a.m.). I'd always taken it at bedtime, so never noticed its drowsy effects until that morning. At least, finally, I'd gotten one benefit promised.

The next year, a friend mentioned the great benefits of SAMe—one of them being sleep[6]—so, like a hobo, I jumped on that passing train. She said two hundred milligrams also worked great for her depressive mood during the winter with a lack of sunshine. (Yes, even Florida has shorter days during our "winter.")

After doing much research, I too started SAMe[7] at two hundred milligrams. They said it could increase natural melatonin production but warned about sleep interference when taken at night. At four hundred milligrams, I found those negative effects of digestive distress they warned about in the form of stomachaches. My friend recommended taking two hundred milligrams in the morning and two hundred more at night. I split them between breakfast and dinner, careful to avoid bedtime doses, and it did the trick. I'd also read you could build tolerance, but after a couple of weeks, when I kicked it back up to four hundred in the morning, the stomachache returned. Having read that most concerns are addressed at the six hundred to sixteen hundred milligram range, I called it quits, being careful to step back down as recommended by professionals.

This too shall pass.

CHAPTER 5

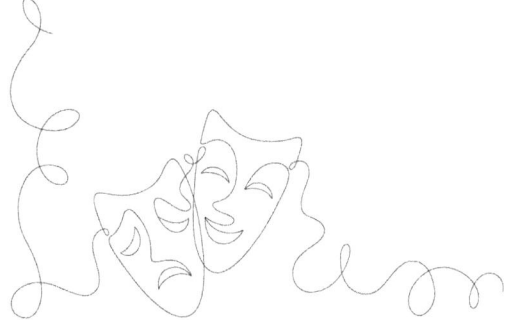

HORMONAL RAGE AND MOOD SWINGS

Hormonal Rage

Nothing to see.

Move it along.

This is where writing this book feels more confessional than informational or instructional. I think most people would rather take it to their grave than discuss the underbelly of hormones: hormonal rage.

My brother, Joe, says I have the Hampton temper. Hampton is my father's side of the family, where the men could show their anger occasionally, but I'm unaware anyone had real anger issues. Besides, I can't dismiss what I've experienced in myself as simply me being a stereotypical redhead or a Hampton.

For instance, one day while I was home for a quick lunch, I found that my mother had left her six-month-old doodle puppy, Buttercup, in the large crate, just in case of a mishap. It would have been easier if she'd had her accident on the tile floor. One wipe and down with a flush. However, the puppy pooped in the crate and then sat in it. When I went to let her out, I saw poop matted under her curly-haired tail. I should've turned the hose on her to remove the mess, but I wasn't thinking clearly. I tried using toilet paper but it made little difference. I returned Buttercup to her crate for quarantine.

The frustration rose.

When I reached into my skinny pantry for a poop bag to use as a glove, my shoulder knocked against the doorjamb.

Pain seared.

At the moment, about four years of dealing with the pantry's puny opening, insufficient time for lunch, sleep deprivation, and dealing with literal crap all collided. Normally, I would've rubbed my shoulder and wished for a larger pantry again. But with the hormonal storm raging inside, I took the door and yanked. Hard. The door fell to the tile floor with a crack.

If the door will not serve my needs, then it must GO! I thought to myself. And with the rage still brewing inside of me, I lifted one end of the downed door and slammed it back down with as great a force as I could muster. The reverberating sound waves hit the weak shelf in the next room. My ears rang with a crash in the croffice, the dual-purpose craft room and office—it's my word and you'll have to pay me a nickel each time you use it.

I peeked around the corner to find the shattered remains of my grandmother's crystal bell glimmering in the daylight. Grief replaced the fury when my heart sank as I swept the shards.

In front of my fallen enemy, I called my brother. "Joe, I ripped the pantry door off the wall."

His voice, full of calmness, offered instruction like a flight attendant on a plane going down: "Just push the metal peg at the top, and it should go back into place. Those doors pop off all the time."

Hormonal Rage and Mood Swings

"No, you don't understand. I *ripped* it off." I recounted the previous five minutes' activities in all their glory.

His laughter overrode my retelling of the event. Finally, he calmed down and offered to come over after work to check it out.

In the evening when I returned from work, my mother had a quite different reaction. "I guess you'll think twice before doing something like that again."

"Seriously? If thinking were a part of this, I would not have done it in the first place." I quelled the new storm threatening inside me.

My whole life, I'd wondered about the people whose tempers had gotten the best of them and cost them dearly in replacement expenditures for tangible items or loss of freedom due to hurting others. For example, in high school, a classmate who found out her boyfriend had cheated on her punched the bathroom tile wall and broke her hand. A few days later, she found the gal he cheated with and beat her into a sticker bush with the freshly set arm cast. In the eighties, a school fight wouldn't normally land you in jail.

I remained vigilant and kept on her good side. I also remember thinking how stupid it was to hurt yourself out of anger. Let alone hurt someone else. Besides, the boyfriend deserved it more than the one he cheated with, but she could've just walked away from it all.

During my life, I've purposed to do better than spiraling out of control; I've never destroyed things or hurt people out of anger.

Then there were hormones. And a lack of sleep. A perfect storm.

One day, I ran an errand for work. They liked to wait until the last minute before telling me I needed to deliver something before closing time—usually at a governmental office, and agency workers don't linger one extra second at the end of the day. I headed out after a flurry of preparations with no slack in my schedule. After several red lights and a slowpoke, I realized my arrival would be too late.

In the moment, I took it out on my sunglasses—my favorite sunglasses. They crunched in my hands before I flung them down to the far corner of the passenger floorboard. Regret set in and I reached for them, but they proved to be a bit hard to grab as I drove down the highway.

The frustration rose again.

When I finally managed to seize them, after a near-death experience, they had little damage, so I made sure they weren't wearable. Ever. Again. "If sunglasses won't make themselves accessible, then they must *go!*"

A great sorrow settled in the land at the death of those shades. They were perfect—not too heavy, the right tint, and fit me well. I have yet to find another pair like them at the discount stores. Breaking them made no sense, I know, but at the moment only anger and frustration prevailed.

Tip: Buy sunglasses from the eye doctor for clearer lenses and overall better quality, but keep them out of the sun and the heat of the vehicles in summer, or they'll warp.

The great sorrow is a joke, but a plethora of emotions followed the hormonal rage incidents. It's a roller coaster of emotions from disbelief to regret and a sprinkle of shame and embarrassment. I can't explain it for the life of me apart from The Change.

The rage never happened before my mid-forties. I've had numerous occurrences that didn't involve breaking things. Now, there's screaming that leaves my throat sore and plenty of crying out to God to fix me or calm the storm. Thankfully, there aren't witnesses to these events. My mother may have been right. If I let my freak flag fly when I'm alone but not with others, perhaps I could control it. Possibly, if I caught it right at the beginning.

Hormonal Rage and Mood Swings

Those instances happened when several things went wrong all at the same time or one annoying thing repeated in a short amount of time. The last one I can recall involved trying to get out of the car. Simple enough on a normal day, but I have a certain personality quirk: I have to get groceries, laundry, or shopping bags all in one trip. It doesn't matter what it is; I always think I can get it all, so I don't have to go back for a second trip.

Who has time for that?

Ordinarily, I do, but time's not the point. It's the challenge, trial, and test, but it's simply an inconvenience to go back again. Therefore, I persist in making myself miserable, like the fateful morning I pulled up to the office. I placed the purse straps over my right shoulder and grabbed my travel mug and the papers I needed to bring to my desk.

Before I could open the door, I spotted a slip of paper lying under my purse and put the other papers back down. I moved the travel mug to my left hand, slung the purse handles back on my shoulder, and took the documents with my right hand. Then I realized I needed the deposit receipt in my left hand with the travel mug so it wouldn't wrinkle. I moved the small square appointment reminder into my left hand with the mug and receipt.

Ready.

Not quite. I forgot to turn off the car. Both hands full made the ignition hard to reach, but I managed. Mindful of not spilling the mug, I carefully pulled at the door handle. Success. Then I spied the office keys in the door's pull cubby. I tried to reach them with my left hand. The reminder slip escaped as did my purse straps. Again.

For the past decade, pick-it-up-and-put-it-down has become the theme of my life. I'd done it this one particular morning too. I'd returned the papers and purse to the passenger seat and the mug to the cup holder. With my foot dangling out the door, I trapped the reminder and snatched it up before the wind caught it. At that point, I realized I hadn't put the windshield shade in place. With the task accomplished, I grabbed the keys and loaded myself up again.

I pushed the door open against gravity in the upward-sloped parking lot and dropped the keys. The door slammed into me as I leaned out. The coffee sloshed and that's when I lost it. It wasn't pretty, but nothing broke. With no one else at the office yet, there were no witnesses, certain the neighbors couldn't hear my screams through the closed doors and windows.

Testimony, gloriously intact.

Estrogen levels start to drop reducing serotonin levels, creating an imbalance of emotions. Many women experience mood swings during The Change.

Tip: Doctors indicate that the worse your premenstrual (PMS) symptoms were, the more likely you are to have more extreme symptoms during menopause.

It hardly seems fair!

If misery does indeed love company, then I'm in good company. Almost a quarter of women going through The Change experience these mood swings in the form of depression, anger, and anxiety. Most of them mention irritability as their first symptom, especially for those who did not have a regular period due to a partial hysterectomy or medications. Depression affects one in five. Anxiety and panic attacks can get worse or happen for the first time. Women can find themselves crying over commercials, songs, or situations that didn't bother them before. Insomnia can affect up to half of all women during menopause.

> **Emotional Symptoms of Menopause Mood Swings**[1]
>
> **"Irritability:** Up to 70 percent of women describe irritability as their main emotional problem during the early stages of the menopausal transition. They find themselves less tolerant and more easily annoyed at things that did not bother them before.
>
> **Depression:** Depression is a more common and serious emotional side effect of menopause. It affects up to 1 out of every 5 women as they progress through menopause.
>
> **Anxiety:** Many women experience tension, nervousness, worry, and panic attacks during menopause. Some may find their anxiety getting worse while others may develop it for the first time.
>
> **Crying episodes and feeling weepy:** This tendency can become more pronounced in menopausal women, as they find themselves weeping over incidents that might not have mattered much before. However, tears can reduce stress as they allow people to release pent-up feelings.
>
> **Insomnia:** Insomnia can contribute to mood swings, as it interferes with day-to-day functioning. It is common during menopause, affecting 40-50 percent of women."

Most people without proper sleep tend to be a little cranky; now up the ante with hormones going awry.

The common opinion indicates a thoughtful approach to hormonal rage: pay attention to what sets you off, see if there's a pattern, and try to avoid it if possible.

Easier said than done, I know. I know. As my boss likes to say, "Sounds good if you say it really fast."

Though I've avoided public outbursts in the past, sometimes I can feel it coming on when I'm around other people. If I'm at home with Dean, he can hear me amping up. He encourages me to walk away from whatever task is sending me over the edge. I will return to it later, or he'll finish my task. Mostly, it's paying attention to the rising anger, then stopping when you're not too far behind, cutting your losses.

You can seek professional help from a reputable mental health counselor to gain tools to help you cope with the rage scenarios and mitigate the damage. Changes in your diet and exercise can also help. (See chapter 2, "Estrogen Overload.")

Mood Swings

Mood swings can affect up to a quarter of women. Like any of the menopause symptoms, most women don't suffer the extreme hormonal conditions, but you probably know someone who does (even if they're not talking about it).

Did you check off most of the list from Emotional Symptoms of Menopause Mood Swings? I did too. My fuse is shorter these days, but I blamed it on the last item on the list: insomnia. I'm not usually an emotional person, but I've cried at more movies, television shows, and commercials in the past eight years, than in the previous forty years. I've always been a little tightly wound, so I wouldn't have guessed anxiety as a menopause cohort.

The dark cloud of depression hasn't kept me company since my awkward school days, and thankfully, it's not one of the emotional problems I suffer from now. For the extreme cases of anxiety and depression, mental health counseling can benefit those suffering.

Aerobic exercise can help lessen the severity of many menopause symptoms. Two to three hours per week can make a difference, but for those over forty, consider high-intensity interval training (HIIT) paired with strength training (weights or resistance bands). Try varying every other day: three days a week for aerobics

Hormonal Rage and Mood Swings

with two days of strength training in between those. You'll also get more from a brisk walk than from a run.

 Tip: You can build up slowly. Make a goal of starting the aerobics at twenty minutes three times per week. Then increase your aerobics until you hit an hour a day. (You can break it into smaller segments, for example a thirty-minute brisk walk in the morning and again after dinner—smaller segments see better results for the over-fifty gals.) Once you've got it down, mix in the strength training in between the aerobics days.

As always, talk to your doctor before trying a new exercise regimen and about your symptoms if diet and exercise don't improve your condition.

CHAPTER 6

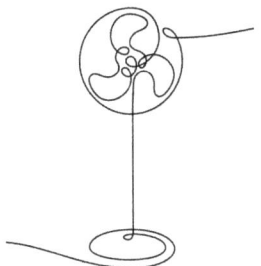

HOT FLASHES AND NIGHT SWEATS

Hot Flashes

Life in Florida revolves around air-conditioning and shade. If we can find a shady parking spot, we'll walk from Goofy's parking lot at Disney to the front door of any store or restaurant, even without a tram. And God forbid the AC goes out at home, work, or in the strategically parked car!

Five years of hot flashes passed, and I blamed the AC units.

All of them.

Everywhere I went.

But it's because the ACs at home, work, and in my car needed attention, and I didn't have a clue what a hot flash was. I had a general idea, but not specifically, until one fateful night.

A couple of months before Dean and I married at fifty, the first time for both of us, we had dinner with friends. We chatted as we sat around their kitchen table. Then the husband teased about his wife's "crazy pills."

Hot Mess Express

My mind scrambled to imagine what private horror she'd been living in. I'd thought I knew her well enough.

Ever the open book, my face must have shown it, because our hostess said, "He's talking about my hormone pills."

Her husband belly laughed. "I don't care what they are, but you were crazy before and now you aren't. They're crazy pills."

"What are they for?" I asked her. "If you don't mind me asking."

"I was a little emotional and irritable, not to mention those hot flashes."

I don't know why I connected my condition to it, but it had to all be a coincidence at only forty-nine years old. I asked anyway, "Can you describe the hot flashes? And don't spare any details."

She gave a description, and bells went off in my head.

"Oh, good grief. I might have those too. I just thought the AC had broken everywhere I went for the past five years!" The room erupted in laughter at my expense.

She said, "Well, the pills helped me tons. You should keep a hot flash log, so you have something to show your doctor."

 Tip: Make a hot flash log, noting each time and duration, so your doctor has a reference when you share your symptoms with him or her.

She gave me the best advice I'd ever received. I started the log. I made a note every time I had a hot flash. It's strange how, when you pay attention, the problem seems more prevalent.

It reminded me of the time I drove from California to Kansas with my mother. We'd only made it from Laguna Beach to Needles, California, before the thermostat stopped working and our radiator overheated. And just like me, the car wasn't to the age you'd expect it to overheat.

My upper back and neck warmed until it felt like someone had turned on a heating pad—on the highest setting. Whatever chair or couch I sat in became intolerable as my body heated the material too. I had to lean forward. The heat localized in my core, mostly the upper back. As I watched the clock, I cooled again within three to five minutes.

Interesting.

Not unbearable, but the discomfort definitely took me out of whatever task of the moment. Even with a light shirt, I had to move my long hair from my neck and back. I either held it up for the duration or swept it to the side and down the front. Common symptoms include

- A sudden feeling of warmth spreading through your chest, neck, and face
- A flushed appearance with red, blotchy skin
- Rapid heartbeat
- Perspiration, mostly on your upper body
- A chilled feeling as the hot flash lets up
- Feelings of anxiety[1]

Hot flashes can occur almost daily or several times an hour. They occur for an average of seven years and, in some women, can occur for more than ten years.[2]

Oh boy.

My younger age and lack of perspiration were just a couple of reasons why I found it hard to jump to a hot-flash conclusion to explain my misery. But as I completed my scientific self-study, I determined I'd had an average of seventeen hot flashes per day. The log included only the incidents I remembered to make note of during waking hours.

Hot Mess Express

"Feel my back. It's on fire," I begged Dean or my mother or whoever heard me when it happened. They were not fans of the request, but I just wanted to know if it felt as hot on the outside to them as it did on the inside to me. On the rare occasion someone agreed, they said it felt weirdly hot.

Confirmation.

Not crazy.

As I continued to pay attention to the hot flashes, they became more tolerable. If you know torture will only last a little while, it's easier to endure.

With an appointment scheduled, I continued to log the episodes for the next month. In the meantime, I went to the health food store for one last shot at "natural" relief.

The gentleman at the store sat with me and asked questions for about half an hour. I let him know I didn't want prescription drugs. I went through the list of things I'd already tried, including the (bioidentical) estrogen estriol topical cream, which I experimented with after the scrapbook ladies first suggested my sleep problem might be menopause. I told him he had one shot at this, and then I'd ask the doctor for help. He led me to a product with black cohosh. He said some women have found relief with it from hot flashes. After a month of taking the OTC product, I found no reprieve and went to my doctor's appointment.

My primary care physician listened to me and examined my log. I left with a prescription for Prempro, a mix of estrogen and progestin (mimics progesterone). She mentioned I could only safely take them for about three years without an increase in cancer risks.

"But it should be enough to get you through this."

If the time comes and the hot flashes persist, I have a list of other things I might try.

Within two weeks of incorporating Prempro into my bedtime routine, the hot flashes alleviated—mostly. She'd put me on the lowest dose, which knocked the hot flashes down from seventeen per day to one every two weeks or so. After a year, I started to wonder if the full dose might have a positive effect on my sleep, whereas the low dose did not. She gave me three months to see.

It did not.

I returned to the lower dose, and the hot flashes increased to a few per week. Nevertheless, they were much better than seventeen per day.

Dean expressed his gratitude for my crazy pills, which kicked in just in time for our beach wedding.

But after two years, the hot flashes returned to a few every day. Though I had my share of hot flashes, I did not suffer the intense sweating usually accompanying them. When they came at night and woke me, I'd ridden them out and gone back to sleep. Others endure something much worse.

Hot Flash Tech Remedies

- The EMBR Wave Bracelet—a battery-powered bracelet that acts as a thermostat. It's "like an ice cube on your wrist" or "like cupping your hands around a hot drink."[3]
- The Hot Flash Pillow—like a long ice pack with a sleeve
- Acupressure Bracelet—These come in many styles and are sold by many companies. A quick Google search will find them for you.
- Menopod—the ad says, "No More Cursing." The tech looks like a computer mouse you hold to the back of your neck when you overheat.

Night Sweats

More than two-thirds of women experience hot flashes and night sweats. Up to a third of those undergo severe symptoms, often enough to soak through clothing and bedding to the point where they need to be changed.[4]

The sweating is your body trying to regulate and cool off after the blood vessels flush with blood (vasodilation). Some doctors speculate the cause is sensitive skin cells. Others think a brain chemical imbalance—"differences in levels of the hormone leptin, which is produced by fat cells, and a drop in blood sugar may play a role in hot flashes."[5]

There may be choices you can make to bring about changes in how often you experience hot flashes and night sweats.

- **Exercise**—inconclusive studies suggest exercise may reduce the frequency of hot flashes.
- **Smoking**—"One study found that heavy smokers were four times more likely to have hot flashes than women who never smoked."
- **Temperature**—use a fan or crank the air conditioner.
- **Cool drinks**—sip on a cold water or decaf iced tea; drink lots of fluids.
- **Triggers**—"alcohol, caffeine, and spicy foods may trigger hot flashes."
- **Relaxation**—"The stress hormone cortisol may make women more sensitive to hot flashes. . . . Take some deep belly breaths when you feel stressed."
- **Diet and Supplements**—Adding OTC supplements like DHEA-dehydroepiandrosterone, dong quai, ginseng, kava, red clover, or soy (soybeans, tofu, tempeh, or miso) to your diet may help, but there are no conclusive studies to prove any real benefits.
- **Medications**—if symptoms persist and interfere with your quality of life, talk to your doctor to see if hormone replacement therapy or antidepressants may help.[6]

Hot Flashes and Night Sweats

The number of women suffering from hot flashes and night sweats may be as much as 85 percent.[7] Doctors recommend trying lifestyle changes like those listed above for at least three months before resorting to prescription medications. You can also try the following doctor-recommended suggestions:

Cool showers—take cool showers during the day and at bedtime

Cold water on wrists—during a hot flash, run cold water over your wrist

Healthy weight—hot flashes can be more frequent and intense for overweight or obese women

OTC supplements—phytoestrogens and black cohosh[8]

Talk to your doctor before adding anything to your diet, even OTC supplements if you're already taking prescriptions, as some herbal supplements can interfere with certain medications.

When I woke during the dark hours from overheating, I didn't perspire, not exactly like night sweats. I only heated up, like a daytime hot flash. When this happened, I couldn't even tolerate skin touching skin. I'd toss the bedding aside and begin to search for the cool spot on the bed. We'd purchased a cooling mattress, but I doubted its ability during those times. Within a few minutes, it did pass and I could drift back off to sleep. I eventually bought a cooling pillow made for toddlers to stick between my legs, which helped a lot.

My heart goes out to those who must change their soaked pajamas before going back to sleep. I know some who had to change the bedding too. Laundry overload!

Keep in mind this will not last forever.

This too shall pass.

CHAPTER 7

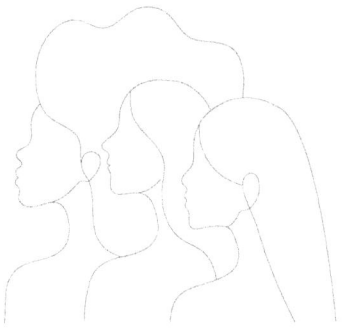

HAIR

My Head—Hair Color

In my mid-to-late thirties, I noticed my hair looking a little dull and lifeless. I had flashbacks to a movie I watched as a child—I couldn't have been more than twelve—a Western with an old lady in her Old West garb, resembling Granny from *The Beverly Hillbillies.*

She had red hair like mine, but mostly gray—not a good look; not glamorous by any means. Not like women with dark hair that turns salt and pepper. Not gorgeous silver, just bland.

When I commented on her hair color, my mother said, "You'll look just like her, because you have red hair too."

She teased, maybe, but it stuck with me. Over the years, I'd noticed that women with darker hair seemed to gray more gracefully. Some were even quite stunning with streaks of gray washing through their darker tresses. Blondes seemed to blend well, too, making it hard to notice the change.

But redheads? We need help. (I have a friend who says brunettes need help too!)

As with blondes, the graying is subtle with redheads; it just looks dull. I don't know how long it'd been going on with me when I finally noticed the drabness.

Some say graying is predetermined by genetics; others claim hormones, illness, and environment can all play their part. I'm not sure of the cause, but my melanocyte stem cells are getting jammed between developing hair follicle compartments. In other words, my protein pigments aren't making red so much anymore.[1]

The next time I saw my brutally honest mother, I asked if she'd noticed the lackluster locks.

"Your brother and I were just talking about that."

My eyes widened.

Partly because of my military family background, my mother instilled in me at a very young age the practice of making myself presentable daily. She taught me to dress right for any occasion and presented me with mascara during my freshman year of high school. I've seldom been without proper clothes, hair, and makeup since and have always tried to look my best.

The words of a friend's mother still buzzed in my brain, "I only went to the grocery store once without my makeup, and don't you know, it's when I ran into everyone I've ever known."

My mother and brother, who'd loved to tease me about anything and everything Sally, did not provide any input on the matter, which stunned me.

"When were you going to say something to me about it?"

"Don't be so dramatic. Our conversation happened only a few days ago."

Small mercies.

She quickly suggested I start hitting the bottle. I asked what brand she used and immediately went to Walmart. The choices for redheads were far fewer than other hair colors, but given my propensity toward decision paralysis, maybe that was a good thing.

Hair

One day before the great dimming of my red crown, someone's child called my attention after church in the lobby. "Why do they call it red hair? It's not the color of a fire engine," the seven-year-old asked.

True.

I had heard years ago that many fire departments have now turned to chartreuse—the fluorescent greenish-yellow—because it's the last color you see before dark, giving them more visibility than the quickly fading red as they race to the next emergency.[2] I resisted educating him on this fact. No, I replied instead, "What would you like to call it?"

"I don't know." He pondered for a bit while I came up with a name.

"How about Burnt Cinnamon Amber?" Half hoping this would dissuade him and I could get on with my day, it worked. We both agreed it would be better than the generic red.

But neither Clairol, Garnier, L'Oréal, nor the others had Burnt Cinnamon Amber. They carried vague names or simply numbers. Not having a medium red, I decided on strawberry blonde rather than auburn and went for the cheapest box, Revlon Colorsilk.

It worked great for a couple of years. Then, without any reason whatsoever, I threw all caution to the wind and switched to another brand. I'd seen a commercial about a retail brand's oil-based color rather than the "harsh chemicals." My hair went flat and my frustration inflated.

Mom gave me her hairdresser's information. She is probably the best colorist around and also gave me a great cut. The coloring helped bring back some shine, but I discovered a product in the ethnic hair care section: Smooth 'n Shine polisher. I use it sparingly to avoid looking too oily—just two fine mist spritzes. I get so many compliments on the shine now, or did until COVID-19 when the product disappeared from store shelves. Four years later, I found it online for triple the price. I might treat myself one day but not for fourteen dollars.

I'd used Mom's gal for more than five years until she decided she didn't want to do hair anymore. If only she'd said something before it started showing in her work.

Insisting on a professional stylist, I tried different hairdressers before landing with a lady from church. The shop she works out of is a block over from my office. Win-win. I've been with her for more than five years now. She had to hear all about the sleep issue and my trials with the VA. I shared how I met Dean and asked her to do my wedding hair, but she doesn't work evenings or weekends. (Good for her!)

She colors my hair, and then eight weeks later, I return. Between appointments, around the four-week mark, the grays reappear. New gray hairs appear mostly in my part and the hairline around my face, especially by my cheekbones. I tried coloring shampoo at first but then realized it only worked on hair strands with color, not grays. I'm sure the root coloring sprays work fine, but I couldn't find one Burnt Cinnamon Amber or anything close.

In my search for a root touch-up, I stumbled upon a powder close to my hair color: Protégé CoverAge. It looks like a blush compact. You apply it at the points of concern with the brush provided, and voilà, you're good to go until the next shampoo. I've experimented with stretching my color appointments to ten weeks, but eight weeks seems to be the sweet spot. Otherwise, I'd used too much powder and painted my whole head.

My Head—The (Thinning) Crown of Glory

Regular haircuts helped with the extra split ends I'd noticed—taming the old-lady frizz, which came with the grays. One day, I asked the stylist if she'd noticed my hair thinning. "I'm sure I can

Hair

see more of my scalp through the hair with harsh overhead lighting, like the office or your salon."

She threw a hand up. "Stop. You are not thinning." At my insistence, she stooped next to me to see the reflection from my vantage point. "I don't see it." She straightened and resumed mixing the colors in a bowl.

Looking at her twentysomething locks, I huffed and continued. "I've been using the shampoo and conditioner for visibly thinning hair for the past two years but haven't seen any difference." I pointed to the expensive bottles on the shelves next to her station. "I've even tried an Amazon-Choice brand, but neither worked."

Rolling her eyes in her wrinkle-free head, she said, "Because you're not thinning."

"But you've only known me for a while. You never saw it before." I messed with my hair to try to prove my point. "It's thinning and the individual strands are skinner! It never really came back after my mishap with an oil-based color I got at the grocery store, which is why I ended up coming to you in the first place, if you remember."

She assured me I imagined my head's glaring scalp, but I knew better.

Growing up, we teased my balding father about his *wavy hair*, "It's waving goodbye to your head." Now I had his receding hairline.

One day I had an itch on the back of my head. I scratched and noticed how much thicker my hair seemed at the base of my head compared to the top.

Confirmation of thinning.

The Bible refers to a woman's hair as her glory, or her pride and joy. It's her cover. My solution-finding intensity increased.

Biotin seemed to be an internet consensus, so when some of my writer friends also suggested it for hair growth, I added it to my morning regimen. Though I didn't notice any improvement in hair or skin, it did strengthen my nails, so I kept taking the supplement.

As I planned my wedding at fifty, I stopped by the county parks office to reserve and pay for a beach pavilion. The woman who helped me seemed to be a good decade older, yet her graying hair remained thick. Genetics? Jealousy overcame me.

"Your hair is gorgeous," I told her.

She smiled. "Thanks. At my request, my boyfriend bought me one of those $100-per-month hair systems, but I think it's the prenatal vitamins I take."

"You can take those without bad side effects even though you're not pregnant?"

With a wave of her hand, she said, "I've checked with my doctor, and he assured me."

I gave those horse-pill excuses for vitamins the same nine months to work in me, just as long as an expectant mother would give them. But by the time I'd long since given birth, I took note of the same sad state of my head. The prenatal vitamins with biotin showed no difference compared to the plain biotin supplements.

Eventually, I decided to up my game and get serious about my father's reflection in my mirror.

On the internet, of course, I waded through a multitude of bad reviews on any of the hair "systems," even those with infomercials. I settled on a generic version of Rogaine for women sold under Walmart's Equate label, Hair Regrowth Treatment for Women. I ordered a three-month supply online and decided to give it the full three months for any improvement.

With little hope and fingers no longer crossed, I perceived a noticeable difference. After only a month and a half, I no longer felt self-conscious about my diminishing mane. I had new growth, which amazed my hairdresser, leaving me glowing in I-told-you-so

Hair

righteousness. I didn't suspect it would grow hair that never existed, but it seemed to bring back what used to be there—mostly.

If you get nothing else from this book, and it applies to you, try this product. You have to use it twice daily. A dropper measures the clear liquid, which dries within a few minutes.

A word of caution: since my hairdresser instructed me to wash my hair only twice weekly, the hairspray builds up and can get a little sticky when this product is first applied, but it's fine after it dries. One reviewer stated it turned to paste with her hair products. I get what she's saying. But, are you kidding me? Bald versus a little sticky until it dries—no contest.

> **Tip:** Apply the product directly to the scalp and massage in with small circles to avoid spreading to hair strands. This should help with the sticky issue.

Another reviewer wrote that if you stop using the product, you will lose all the hair growth you gained. No big deal. I'm hedging my bets on a permanent fix from the scientific community within the next decade. Look, you have to brush your teeth twice a day anyway, so do this at the same time. Seriously, thirty seconds, and you're done.

It's a high reward and low cost—nothing to it! I'm not aware of an easier or cheaper fix. And it's worth my husband's teasing, even though Dean sometimes uses a hair color made just for men that keeps some of the gray.

Years ago, I'd heard about the feminine mystique from an older lady at church, not the second-wave feminist book by Betty Friedan but just the idea of leaving it a mystery how we put ourselves together for the day or a night out. So, I tried to be inconspicuous with some of the beautification treatments, especially during our first year of marriage. I'm sure the treatments paled in comparison to Esther's of the Old Testament, but I still tried to maintain the feminine mystique in front of Dean.

I've repeatedly told him, "Trust me; you don't want to see how the sausage is made."

Of course, this gal furthermore tried to hide the realities of having IBS while we dated. One time I ran for the bathroom; "Keep the movie going." But he hit pause on the DVR. I screamed from the bathroom (with no exhaust fan) for him to turn the television volume up. I came out to him shaking a can of Lysol. "Do you need this?" And he still married me.

As hard as I tried to hide the ugly side of my beauty treatments, he caught me using the magic hair potion. "Is that to cover the gray?" He knew I'd recently gone to the salon for the color and cut.

"Yeah. Sure. It's for the 'gray'." I used air quotes, so he couldn't call me a liar. Now he refers to the balding tonic as "Just for Old Ladies." Great.

It takes only thirty seconds, twice daily, but you wouldn't believe the number of times he'd walked in during the application. I don't care anymore. It is what it is. The other day, I made a grocery list with the product on the list. Dean nearly died laughing, because I'd written "Just for Old Ladies" on the paper.

Perfect, he had me calling it that too.

 Tip: Avoid looking like a werewolf by using care when applying the hair growth serum. You might notice extra peach-fuzz hair as I did on my forehead when it ran down numerous times without thoroughly rinsing it.

My Face

Somewhere around forty, I started tweezing more on my eyebrows. With hair now growing above and below the actual eyebrows and sprouting out into the crow's feet, almost daily I find a new rogue hair to tackle.

The tweezing doesn't stop at the eyes. Regretfully, the nose also commands attention. Yes, the hair inside my nose all of a sudden started sprouting. One day my nose tickled. I rubbed it, but it nonetheless continued. As soon as I got to a mirror, I saw the annoying stray hair curling out from inside my nose. I immediately plucked it.

From the men's section, I bought a nose and ear hair shaver. Maybe the clerk assumed I purchased them for a man in my life. I didn't really care. I needed it, but not for the ears. Not yet, and though it's possible, hopefully, never will. Seriously, how much can one woman take?

When I started dating the man the prophecies had foretold (it's OK to laugh here), it had come to pass that the peach fuzz above my lip had morphed into a bit more too. Since I'd only dated once in the past twenty years (besides three blind dates, but those don't count), I didn't give it much thought. But with the first kiss in over two decades potentially looming, the concern over the mustache prompted me to ask my brother about it—since he's a man.

Bad move.

He leaned in to examine the 'stache. He squinted his eyes and crinkled his face only slightly. "I don't think it's any worse than Peanut's."

Peanut is what he lovingly calls his good friend's fifteen-year-old son. I understood and immediately found the time to visit the salon. I didn't make an appointment, and my usual person wasn't there.

One of the other stylists in the back spotted me. She hollered from her station, "Can I help you?"

After I hesitated and decided only women occupied the shop, I yelled past the others, "I'm fixin' to have my first kiss in two decades and I need my mustache waxed."

We all laughed and had a good time at my expense, then she waved me back. "I can do it for you."

Six minutes and five dollars later (plus a two-dollar tip), it felt as smooth as a baby's butt.

However, it took Dean another three weeks to find the right time to knock my socks off, so I tended the garden of my upper lip with tweezers. Looks like the biotin did work on hair growth, just not the hair I had in mind. The process took longer than expected, so I treated myself to new tweezers.

Tip: You don't have to spend a great deal on tweezers, but don't get the cheapest pair. Quality does matter. The pointed tips grip better than the angled ones for single stray hairs.

A wire spring facial hair remover caught my attention, so I bought the product for eighteen dollars. It is in the shape of a wishbone. You twist one end manually while holding it against the area of unwanted hair. Somehow, the contraption proved more painful than tweezing, perhaps from the surprise of not knowing exactly when it would grab another hair.

Then I turned to an As Seen on TV product. It promised painless hair removal. It caused no pain, but that's because it's a shaver, which encourages growth. It also had a light, but I'm using my lighted bathroom to groom myself, not a dark cave.

Years before, I'd tried the stinky cream hair removal to no avail, so I remained apprehensive about trying another in-home hair removal process—perhaps like the stories of childbirth pain you supposedly forget as they place the baby into your arms. Instead, I decided to wax myself.

At Sally's Beauty Supply store, I had them hook me up with an all-purpose soft wax and a hard wax in cans, a can warmer, sticks to apply, and strips for removing. I promptly asked for my namesake discount. No, they wouldn't give me the "Sally" discount—Hampton Inn never gave me the discount either (my maiden name). I joined both rewards programs instead.

With minimal regret, I managed the undertaking. There was a learning curve, like with most new endeavors. A messy learning curve, but I no longer twirl the edges of my mustache like a villain in a *Rocky & Bullwinkle* cartoon.

Tip: My aesthetician has since informed me that if I had asked her to do it, she would not have started me waxing my upper lip. She said it's the one area that never seems to slow or thin, but waxing only strengthens and quickens it. I suspect nose hair to be the same.

My Legs and Toes

If I shaved in the mornings, I had a five-o'clock shadow on my legs by three in the afternoon. Sooner, if I got a shiver. A few years earlier, I'd won $2,000 in laser hair removal at a shop's grand opening. It's supposed to be the perfect solution to unwanted hair, but they warned me it works best on fair skin and dark hair. Though I had the right complexion, they said I'd have limited success with my fair hair. I gave the certificate to someone who fits the bill and continued shaving infrequently—one of the few perks of singleness.

Then Dean came along. With his love language of touch, Dean constantly rubbed my back or shoulders. During those Sunday lunches in our dating months, he would sit next to me and rub my calves. The first time he did this, I had not shaved in a couple of days. I'd worn a long skirt, so I didn't think about it until he went under the material. He whipped his hand out and held it above the table.

"Ouch! You cut me." He dramatized my prickly legs wounding his fingers.

Perfect.

With my lip-waxing success to encourage me, I decided to branch out to my stems. I'd used the all-purpose wax. When it melted in the can, I dipped a stick and brought it to my leg. I tried to be careful, but strings of wax floated to the counter, the floor, and the towel I'd set out. There were tears. Tears from the pain and tears from the frustration with the mess. After managing only a couple of strips, I gave up.

That's what money is for: paying someone else to make or clean a mess or manage the chores too painful to do yourself. I could not have done my armpits, let alone the bikini area.

The cosmetologist at the salon set an appointment for a month out, so all the hairs could grow long enough. By then I could feel the breeze waving the hairs on my legs. I'd decided she could do the armpits too. I had so much hair. I felt like a hippie.

It turned out I knew the cosmetologist from a financial class I facilitated a few years earlier. We chatted a bit as she led me to a private room with a heated pad on a covered massage bed. Relaxing music played in the background. She also had a nervous giggle if I cried out as she quickly ripped the hairs from their follicles. It's a good thing I already knew her.

I learned to internalize my suffering.

Hair

The tops of my feet, or instep, started growing hair several years ago, along with my toes. As a fair-skinned ginger, my hair is light. Very light. Most people didn't notice the hair unless the sun shone—in Florida. I didn't want to discourage any potential future husband from rubbing my hobbit feet.

Dean loves my feet. "Your toes are squared off making them look like Fred Flintstone's." He even told some of his family members how cute my feet were. They were not as amused.

The comparison rang odd with me and I told him he'd better not have a sick foot fetish. "If I find jars of feet in your place, I'm outta here."

Forty minutes later at the salon, after letting Sabrina do my feet, too, the torture session ended with my legs, upper lip, and pits hairless. Mostly.

The internet community recommended waxing every four to six weeks, but I'm on the short side thanks to either my naturally quick hair growth or biotin. I laid off the biotin to see. Months later, my nails broke more easily, but my hair still grew quickly. I'm leaning toward genetics.

After only a couple of years, I had much less hair, but the "success" of waxing wasn't quite as fruitful as with other women. Because my hair grows quickly, I only enjoy about a week of smooth skin before new growth starts. Others reported about two weeks and slowed growth, so they can go up to six weeks between treatments. My leg hairs often break during removal, so they're a little prickly, which is probably why I don't get the hair-free two weeks others enjoy.

Overall, I'd recommend waxing and wish I'd started decades ago. I might be brave enough to do my legs again one day, but armpits and the bikini line are out of the question.

The Bikini Area

The bikini area is the most sensitive part of the body for waxing, and because of that, it's the most difficult area to wax yourself. During the COVID-19 months (. . . and months), my aesthetician, who specializes in skin, shut down for more than six months. Since I already had the supplies on hand, I ventured into this arena of self-torture. With the bikini wax, I attempted to keep up the grooming standards to which my husband had become accustomed.

What normally took her twenty minutes of speed torture took me an hour and a half. After the Brazilian soft wax heated for forty minutes, I spread out a wax-dedicated towel and the rest of the supplies.

I warned Dean not to come in; he didn't need to see how the sausage was made. Nevertheless, each time, in a rush to finally end the agony, I'd spread the wax too thin and over too much area. Not thinking I had enough zest left in me to rip any more hair from my nether region, I almost called out for help. Instead, I'd taken a few minutes, wiped the sweat from my brow and upper lip, and breathed deeply—taking twice as long to exhale—until I'd mustered enough courage to finish the job.

Each time, I swore I'd never do it again, and I spent the next twenty minutes cleaning wax off of every surface within a six-foot radius. Two months after each session, I found myself half-naked on the bathroom floor, warning Dean not to come in and praying businesses would return to normal because waxing is not a pain easily self-administered.

 Tip: The bikini area can get ingrown hairs. Sometimes, they're just below the surface and you can scratch the skin lightly to break them free. Other times, they form a cyst under

> the skin. Do not break the skin or squeeze it like a pimple, which can cause infection and scarring. I use Adult Acnomel zit cream to help dry them up and Tend Skin to unclog the pores and help the hairs break through. It can take months for the cyst to completely disappear.

The Rest of My Body

At twenty-seven, I'd first experienced a crazy rogue hair growing. In Germany, in 1995, during my last year of enlistment in the army, I happened to be one of the only two junior enlisted females on our Terrain Analyst Team (MOS 81Q). We did map interpretation for cross-country troop movement.

We drew the travel routes for make-believe scenarios for army field exercises. Playing war. In our office, we had large tables pushed together to spread out the maps. We used clear overlays to depict our suggestions for routes to the higher-ups. As we created our overlays, we'd sprawl out on top of the large map tables.

One day, in such close quarters, one of the guys jumped back off the tables and away from me as if I had a contagion and said, "Eww, what's that?" He pointed at me in front of about seven others in the room.

What he could be talking about? I jerked backward. A booger? Did I drool again due to my 1985 jaw surgery nerve damage?

"You have a long hair coming out of your chin!"

Mortified, I ran for the latrine. I searched my reflection in the mirror, grappled for said hair, and almost missed it. The light in the office must've been just right. Or just wrong. How could I have never noticed it before? The rogue hair had to be at least an inch long. I'd missed it because I'd never looked for it.

Why would I be looking for a granny hair at twenty-seven years old?

Why did it have to be a male coworker who noticed my first rogue hair? I've tweezed it enough after two decades, and now it no longer returns. I'm waiting for the other rogue hairs to give up too. I have one on my arm and one on my lower back, which I've fought for years. Have you ever tried to tweeze something you can't see or pull a muscle trying to get to?

Not fun.

Two more have surfaced since marrying Dean. They're on each inner thigh, past where I wax, just above my knees. I cringed at the thought of Dean finding one before I discovered and plucked it. I didn't want to hear Sasquatch jokes for the rest of my life.

Too late. Almost thirty years after the first rogue chin hair, Dean and I got into his car after chatting in the parking lot with a small group after church. When the door closed, he informed me of my wild chin hairs. Once home, I went for the ten-times magnification mirror, and sure enough. How had I missed those? I'd gotten a little slack on the daily taming. I thought it would be easier to sit for twenty minutes once or twice a month instead of obsessing every morning. Wrong, again.

Sometimes, when Dean catches me tweezing, he'll say, "Oh, good. NASA called and said they were getting interference with the satellites."

Good times.

Recently, I caught him tweezing his brows before church. "Oh, good. The neighbors were concerned those hairs would knock the kids off their bikes." Ah, yes . . . good for the goose . . . good for the gander.

My eyebrows got a bit out of control, too, but I've pretty much stuck to tweezing. Recently, experts warned that tweezing to get pencil-thin eyebrows leads to hair not growing back. Can't wait.

If only.

Tip: Brazilian hard wax attaches mostly to the hair and is good for tender areas, like the bikini area. It has to set before you can pull it up. Soft wax adheres more to the skin, which is good for the legs and armpits. Applied with a flat wooden stick, you can remove the wax with cloth-like strips made for hair removal.

CHAPTER 8

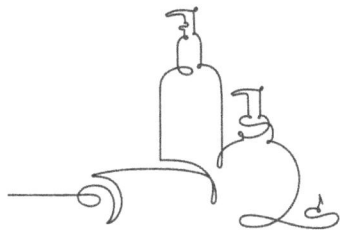

SKIN

Dry Skin

Dry, itchy skin?

Sounds like a commercial.

Maybe dryness has always been the case for you, but for me, it's just starting. I think. I've been using face lotion day and night, and body lotion on the rest after my showers since my twenties.

Ever since my mother became a Revlon and Ultima II representative in the eighties, she impressed upon me the importance of a good face lotion. Washing each night before bedtime added to the nighttime routine she taught me, but it didn't stick. I don't wear foundation, so I don't feel like it's a big deal, but don't report me to one of those skincare tyrants. I lazily use makeup remover wipes each morning, and I use special face soap when I wash my hair in the shower two days a week.

I'm reminded of an episode of *Everybody Loves Raymond*. Debra did her bedtime routine as the couple got ready for bed, and

Raymond lamented growing older—his life half over already. She accused him of having a ridiculous pity party. Her face contorted, and with no sympathy, she explained why she put lotion on her elbows. While scolding him, she stated she didn't have to moisturize in her younger years, but now older, she does.

He remained speechless with fear, as usual, and they went on with the show. I can't remember anything else about the episode, but the elbow scene stuck with me over the years. I didn't understand then why she would need to use lotion in her advancing years. Lately, I've been getting the drift. In a post office conversation with a clerk, he said he could guess my age. I knew I had him with my baby face and girlish figure.

He said, "Turn around."

Flabbergasted, I refused the coarse request.

"I'm not a pervert; I just want to see your elbows," he insisted.

Ever the compliant one, I slowly turned.

He blurted out, "Thirty-five."

Spot on! What witchcraft doth this young man wield?

"Thirty-six, how'd you know? What is it about my elbows?"

"You can do things to look younger, but you cannot do anything to the elbows."

It struck a chord with me. It might also explain the old rule for women over fifty to wear sleeves of at least three-quarters length.

In my twenties, I started with Nivea in a can but moved to St. Ives in a large pump bottle as expenses got tighter after the army. I also switched from Borghese to Clinique for face lotion for the same reason—their Dramatically Different yellow lotion is one of my few splurges in any makeup department.

My elbows got a daily dose of body lotion, but it didn't work. The postman proved correct. I don't know how much is genetics, but my grandmother always had great skin. Her nighttime regimen consisted of a face smeared with Vaseline.

Skin

I watched the pastor's son play a high school basketball game in my early forties. I sat near the family with a friend. The pastor's twelve-year-old daughter said something to me, and while laughing, she grabbed my forearm to steady herself.

In disbelief, she cried out, "Mom, you gotta feel Sally's skin. It's so soft." She continued to touch it until I made her stop.

The question remained if my consistent lotion use made my skin much softer than the average person's. Pastor's daughter seemed to think so.

Fast-forward a decade. Soon after we married, I did the same thing to Dean: laughed and touched his arm—skin as soft as mine. I accused him of being a metrosexual and asked if he used lotion. He said he did not, but I had my doubts. I now know his habits, and I can attest body lotion is not a part of his daily routine. Genetics.

I'd married a man with softer skin than mine.

You can also try castor oil (organic, cold-pressed, hexane free, 100 percent pure) mixed with coconut oil (organic, cold-pressed, hexane free, 100 percent pure—solid form) to thin out the heavy castor oil. Melt the coconut oil in a glass container sitting in hot water (do not boil), then mix even parts and store in a dark bottle with a pump. Ooh la la. What a treat. It's messy but it works. I apply at bedtime. It eventually soaks in, but you might have some ruined jammies and sheets—proceed with caution.

 Tip: Pat the skin dry with a towel after bathing instead of rubbing to help maintain the skin's natural oils. A colder bath or shower can also help preserve oils.

Bugs-Crawling Sensation

I've had longer hair for most of my life. Occasionally, I'd feel loose hair down my shirt. I usually found it clinging to the inside of the top. When I pulled it out, the sensation stopped. Starting in my forties, I went shirt diving for loose hair not there. I kept feeling bugs crawling on my skin.

The sensation of bugs crawling across your skin is called formication, caused by dry and thinning skin. Some say the sensation feels like ants marching on their skin. My mind pictures spiders. You can treat it with OTC allergy meds like Benadryl or Zyrtec. My doctor prescribed Loratadine, which I found in generic form at the store. You can also try lotions like Aveeno, CeraVe, and Eucerin if dry skin is the culprit. But it could also be caused by an iron deficiency, starting or stopping certain drugs, and other medical conditions including fibromyalgia, Parkinson's, and skin cancer. If lotion doesn't do the trick, consult your doctor.

Vaginal Dryness

This is certainly the number-one symptom women don't want to talk about: vaginal dryness. Believe me, I don't want to talk about it either, but what is vaginal dryness? I'm glad you asked. (No, I'm not, but if I can talk about poop, I can talk about this!) You know how you apply lipstick or balm and press your lips together to spread the goo, but instead, they're dry and you don't have any moisturizer? Yeah, it's like that. Dry. Like winter dry. Not too bad daily, but it can be itchy, like any other dry skin.

There is relief with moisturizer, just like most other body parts. There are OTC sprays, lotions, and oils, which are fine for the outer areas. However, doctors recommend using water-based products inside the vagina. Check with your gynecologist for any product they recommend, as some products can mess with your natural vaginal flora (the good bacteria).

Before my partial hysterectomy at forty-seven, I had an overabundance of moisture. My underwear stayed moist. After the surgery, I welcomed the change from a humid jungle to the arid desert—until I got married. We got married in the middle of perimenopause, an adventure for both of us. Since we waited until the wedding night to have sexual intercourse, we were in for a surprise. He would've had an easier time walking through a wall.

    Unprepared, I panicked. He said he'd wait until after a trip to the corner pharmacy the next day, but not me. We'd both had sex before meeting each other, but I'd stopped having sex outside of marriage and had waited over two decades for this honeymoon! Unwilling to wait one more day, I improvised with lotion. I found it better than nothing, but I quickly started a search for something more conducive.

    For general vaginal dryness, you can use a vaginal moisturizer to coat the vaginal cells, keeping them from deteriorating further. It's applied at home with an applicator once every few days. Your body uses what it needs and dispels the rest. It can be quite wet for the first day, so a panty liner is recommended. I have tried this with the Replens my doctor gave me but found the initial abundance of wetness to be uncomfortable and disruptive during my sleep. The next three or four days were much better.

    Frequent sex (one to two times per week) will also help keep the cells healthy—use it or lose it. For painful sex, you can add a vaginal lubricant. Applied on the penis or the vaginal opening, it helps things slide better. Again, try to use water-based products instead of silicone to avoid disrupting the vaginal flora.[1]

    However, my recent VA gynecologist said, "Everything messes with the flora. Having sex messes with the bacteria. Use what works best for you." She also encouraged me to use it every time we have sex to avoid soreness indicative of damage. Are you sore every time? Then lube every time.

The official name for vaginal dryness is postmenopausal vaginal atrophy or genitourinary syndrome of menopause (GSM). It includes

- Vaginal dryness
- Vaginal burning
- Vaginal discharge
- Genital itching
- Burning with urination
- Urgency with urination
- Frequent urination
- Recurrent urinary tract infections
- Urinary incontinence
- Light bleeding after intercourse
- Discomfort with intercourse
- Decreased vaginal lubrication during sexual activity
- Shortening and tightening of the vaginal canal[2]

Another option to help with vaginal dryness is local vaginal estrogen in the form of rings, inserts, and creams. Not the same as hormone replacement therapy, these can be used in addition to BHRT. (Talk to your doctor about trying this therapy.) I settled on the estradiol cream over the others. It is applied with a vaginal insert at bedtime and can thicken the thinned vaginal walls and reduce the symptoms of dryness, itching, and burning. As my vaginal walls thickened, I no longer had the soreness after sex like I did with lubricant alone.

After being absorbed all night, any extra cream passes during my morning bathroom visit, and there are more than twenty hours after application before sex. That is important. You should use caution with vaginal estrogen so your husband doesn't have direct contact. He's likely already struggling with declining testosterone and doesn't need your estrogen. Besides, women don't usually like

Skin

feminine men outside of Anthony Andrews in the must-see 1982 movie *The Scarlet Pimpernel*.

 Tip: There is usually some vaginal estrogen cream left on the applicator. Apply the tiny amount to the urethra to help with occasional coughing and sneezing urinary leak problems.

Crepey Skin

Drier skin is only the tip of the foreboding iceberg. Next on the list are crepey skin and wrinkles. I hadn't paid too much attention to the crepey skin outside the occasional television commercial until Dean mentioned his hands. He's meticulous with the sunscreen while surfing, and even uses the special high-SPF version (made especially for faces) on his hands too. I told him he had crepey skin and looked at the backs of my own hands. Though an eighteen-year-old still stared back at me in the mirror, my hands reflected a woman as old as Dean initially thought me to be.

This is the point where I'd felt like I had crested the hill and started careening down the other side.

The backs of my hands resembled the "before" pictures in a commercial. I didn't mention it to Dean but gave him some of my surplus lotions from the numerous Clinique gift-with-purchase packs I'd accumulated. When it ran out, he bought some face, hand, and body lotion. I told him there was no such thing; they used false advertising. He laughed and showed me the tube, which mentioned all three parts of the body.

But I reiterated, "You can use the same stuff on your face and the backs of your hands. But what's mild enough for the face is not nearly strong enough for the body, and vice versa."

A year and a half later, he bought another tube of the same product. He put it on the backs of his hands as well as on the deepening line on his face. I finally got him with the same joke he kept using on me, "How many tubes of that stuff have you used?"

He turned slowly; his face registered recognition of the turnabout.

I stifled laughter. "When's it gonna start working?"

Bam! I'd waited a year and a half to return that one-liner. Even though he's a notorious sufferer of CanDishItOutButCantTakeIt-itis, he received it well.

Crepey skin can be dealt with by professionals using lasers, retinol creams, ultrasound, and CoolSculpting. Try to avoid overexposure to the sun and remember to cleanse gently and use a moisturizer.[3]

Cracking Heels

Even my feet are starting to show cracks on the heels from dryness, the one beauty step I thought I'd stayed on top of through the years. About fifteen years ago (in my mid-thirties) I attended a friend's home-sales party. Through my church circles of friends, we had lots of them back then for bags, crystal bakeware and dishes, home decorations, and this particular beauty and skincare party. We soaked our feet and then pampered them with a sugar scrub, moisturizing oils, and creams.

My friend said, "I've worn lotion with socks on my feet for years, and I've never had those cracking heels."

In hindsight, she probably had not had her fortieth birthday yet, but the information stuck with me. I applied it and have stayed with it over the years.

Then, I got creative. I switched from the tried-and-true Vaseline to special foot creams. And because I married a Florida-raised man, the air-conditioning is about five degrees higher than I've been

Skin

accustomed to during my single years. Because of the hotter temperature, I gave myself a lotion-and-sock vacation now and then.

Big mistake! When will I learn? If it ain't broke, don't fix it.

This year, I noticed a fissure in both heels—a deep crack. Without treatment, they can become wounds. It would be best if you washed with a nonfoaming hydrating cream or milk cleanser, then moisturize your still-wet feet after each bath or shower. Use products with petrolatum, glycerin, hyaluronic acid, or colloidal oatmeal. Try nonfoaming, liquid formulas.[4]

Tip: I've tried castor oil, and it worked just as good as the petroleum jelly, plus you can use it on the rest of your body. (Mix 50/50 with coconut oil to thin it out.)

Use an exfoliating moisturizer or a foot file, but avoid the cheese-grater type. Twice a week, at the end of my shower, after my feet have soaked, I use a sandpaper-looking file on the small grit side. Now and again, I'll flip it over to the large grit to get a little deeper. Doctors warn not to go too deep with foot files. Cuts and scrapes can cause infection.

If you've waited too long and the cracks are bleeding, try a liquid bandage to seal the wound and keep it clean.

Then, like lemon juice in my foot fissures, a doctor in an article I read said to apply Vaseline to the foot heels and wear cotton socks to bed.[5]

Confirmation. I'd been on the right track all these years. If only I hadn't veered off course. (KISS—Keep It Simple, Sally.) They listed a few OTC products to help heal the cracks: CeraVe Healing Ointment, O'Keeffe's for Healthy Feet Foot Cream, Olive & June Heel Balm, Aveeno Foot Mask, and CeraVe Renewing SA Foot Cream.[6]

If OTC products don't work, see your doctor. You could be missing certain elements in your diet. If it's only dryness, your doctor can prescribe emollients, such as ammonium lactate or urea cream. These should return your skin to a nonreptile condition. Use lotion or Vaseline to maintain.[7]

Passing on the foot creams, I turned to Eucerin with socks at bedtime since the cracks weren't open and sore. It worked great. After only a few weeks, I returned to my grandma's favorite beauty aid, Vaseline.

Veins

My hands show my veins now more than ever. They aren't varicose veins, but with the thinning skin, they are more visible. Everywhere. I even have thick, dark veins showing behind my knees that are sometimes painful. A doctor said they're from trauma: gymnastics, cheerleading, cross-country running and track, aerobics, volleyball, softball, or lugging heavy packs on twelve-mile marches in the army. I couldn't say which for sure—perhaps it's cumulative.

While trying to catch a husband, I allotted a certain amount of funds toward taking care of some of the skin problems that had snuck up on me, including vein treatments called sclerotherapy. I'd already considered doing it before I met Dean, but the relationship gave me the nudge to spend the cash on such a frivolous venture.

"It's an investment," my mother said.

"Sure, that's how I'll justify it." And I did.

Even though a dermatologist would've done those small procedures, I got the feeling from a previous experience that they were more concerned with the task than with appearances. I asked around and found a reputable plastic surgeon.

For the veins, they wouldn't touch the ones behind my knees and said I'd need a phlebologist to make sure it wasn't something more serious. But they went ahead with the sclerotherapy and shot saline into the spider veins on my thighs, which recessed them enough to be less visible. My sister had them in the same spot, but Mom did not, so I assumed they were from smacking my thighs during cheerleading.

My VA doctor assured me the veins behind my knees were nothing to worry about and only surgery, known as varicose vein stripping, would minimize them. She said the procedure included pulling them out like spaghetti.

There are only a few medical reasons for varicose vein stripping:

- Constant pain, throbbing, and tenderness in the legs
- Skin sores and ulcers
- Blood clots
- Bleeding from the veins[8]

Varicose vein stripping may also be done for cosmetic reasons. Like any other serious surgery, it involves anesthesia and incisions, and you'll be off your feet for a few days with a total recovery time of three to four weeks.

The treatment seemed extreme for cosmetic concerns. My veins stopped hurting when I dropped the extra twenty-five pounds, so I haven't done anything else about them.

Bruises

Because of thinning skin, you lose part of the fat insulation that usually protects the blood vessels from injury.[9] Bruises are more apparent. Now, with the sleep issue, I run into doors, desk corners, and coffee tables regularly. I constantly ask myself, "Where'd that bruise come from?" Bruises seem to happen more easily now. They're also prominent, and they stay longer.

My recent clumsiness had become a talking point I'd worked into conversations over the years, so when the time came, people wouldn't think I married an abuser.

Moles, Other Growths, and Skin Cancer

During my high school years, a doctor removed two moles from my face but left a third on my cheek, which always bothered me. He said, "for personality," but it's the wrong kind of personality for a kid in high school. It's now gone—along with some others that had developed on my body.

The one under my high ponytail turned out to be an abscess. The year before, the VA dealt with an abscess on my back, right where the bra connects. The doctor said they don't usually remove them unless they bother the patient or diminish functionality. Since it hurt to lean back, they proceeded: snip, snip, tug, tug, stitch, stitch. They also removed the one on my head because the ponytail's anchoring band rubbed it.

Having known someone with cancer in their thumb, I'm well aware that cancer can materialize anywhere, and time is your enemy when fighting it. Therefore, when you get strange new growths or crusty areas, mention them to your doctor.

So far, so good for me. And I now have a topical medication for those crusty areas of eczema, clobetasol.

Check yourself regularly (use a mirror or ask a loved one for those hard-to-see areas), and record any growth or areas of concern to help you notice when they change.[10] The "ABCDE" guide below is recommended to assist in self-examining any growths.

Follow the "ABCDE" Guide[11]

A = Asymmetry—Common moles are symmetrical. This means that if you draw a line down the center of a mole, the two halves will look the same. Early melanomas are asymmetrical (not symmetrical).

B = Border—Early melanomas often have uneven borders. They may even have scalloped or notched edges.

C = Color—Common moles are usually a single shade of brown or black. Early melanomas are often varied shades of brown, tan, or black. As they progress, red, white, and blue may appear.

D = Diameter—The diameter is the width of a circle across its center. The diameter of a melanoma is usually larger than a mole, though it can be smaller. Early melanomas generally grow to at least the size of a pencil eraser (about ¼-inch across).

E = Evolution—Changes not otherwise described above.

Other Changes to Look For

Sensation—Itching is the most common early symptom. Skin cancers are usually painless, but there can be tenderness and pain.

Size—A mole is suddenly bigger or continues to get bigger.

Spreading color—Melanomas can be a variety of colors, and the color may spread from the edge into the surrounding tissue.

Elevation—A flat or slightly raised mole grows higher very quickly.

Surrounding skin—The skin around a mole becomes red or develops colored blemishes or swelling.

Surface—A mole's surface changes from smooth to scaly, eroding and oozing. A crusty, ulcerated, or bleeding mole is a sign of advanced disease.

"If any of these changes or symptoms appears, make an appointment with your doctor right away. A dermatologist specially trained in skin cancer should be able to recognize a melanoma at its earliest stage."[12]

Being ginger-haired with a peaches-n-cream complexion, I've had numerous sunburns, which has increased my cancer risk. All the fun I had peeling my skin off after a bad burn only makes keeping an eye out for changes now all the more important. A Brown University study found that Caucasian women with at least five of those blistering sunburns during the last half of their teens greatly increased their risk for melanoma and other cancers.[13]

My first bad burn happened in Spain at the tender age of three. My apologetic mother said, "I didn't know. We didn't have sunscreen back then."

Sunburns were a part of my childhood and still are if I'm not careful. At least I didn't put the Hawaiian Tropic or Wesson Oil on my fair skin and then lay out for hours like other gals. I now know to keep an eye on things. An older, fair-complected coworker uses Efudex Cream (Fluorouracil). It treats precancerous and cancerous skin growth by blocking abnormal cell growth.[14]

He uses it once a year on his arms and neck. If you use this pharmaceutical product, do so in the winter when you can wear long sleeves and turtlenecks to cover the angry skin. It looks like a freak show, but not for long.

Age Spots

For a redhead, I have only a smattering of freckles. If I'm careful in the sun and use lots of sunscreen, I'll get just a few more—mostly across the bridge of my nose—during the hot months. Those fade along with summer, but not the age spots. They appear like fat freckles. The first one I saw materialized below my neckline, visible with any open-collared shirt. I used cover-up at first, thinking the spot would eventually fade. It did not.

Skin

Those aren't freckles on the backs of my hands, either. I think my hands have taken the brunt of the menopause effect on my skin. Two on my face joined the ranks. I touch my face too much to worry about foundation unless it's a special occasion, like my wedding. Or so I thought, but when the age spots grew and darkened, I started wearing foundation over concealer to cover them. I had to train myself to stop touching my face—no easy task. What's that about old dogs and new tricks?

Also called liver spots, solar lentigines, and sunspots, they're from spending time in the sun and are more common in light-skinned adults over fifty. Usually found on the face, hands, and upper back, they are not normally dangerous. However, check with your doctor if they are black, getting bigger, not particularly round, not a single color, or bleeding.[15]

(Update: in the time it took me to write this book, four more popped up. Maybe people will assume they're freckles!)

Wrinkles

Just in time for my fiftieth birthday, I decided to tackle my face's wrinkles and age spots. From my catch-a-husband fund, I bought a tube of prescription-strength retinoid, Retin-A. First developed for acne, this vitamin A–based drug may reduce the appearance of fine lines and wrinkles. I've used many OTC products espoused to do the same, but being a medicine-resistant ginger, I have more faith in the ones doctors dole out. Retinoids are also supposed to fade age spots and improve skin color, but it takes six months to a year.[16]

The premixed tube cost ninety-eight dollars, so it seemed like a good idea. And truly, it would've been, but I hit the perfect storm using it. Altogether, it wasn't such a big deal, just bad timing. I'd invited a few people to the house to enjoy a sit-down birthday dinner, for which my mother graciously offered to cook.

That morning, I heated a can of wax to attend to the fuzz on my upper lip and eyebrows, thinking the red skin would fade before guests arrived. It always hurts to some extent. Though I didn't notice additional pain, the burning skin remained a couple of hours later, and the redness hadn't faded.

A shine next to my eyes and at the corners of my mouth where skin used to be drew concern. I asked my mother, who had also tried the waxing that morning, "Is your skin irritated from the waxing?"

"No, I don't think so. Take a look." Her skin remained clear—not red at all.

The raw skin dried and scabbed enough before the party for me to apply cover-up over those areas. When the others arrived, I singled out a friend who'd also tried the retinoid cream and pulled her aside.

"Look at my face. I waxed this morning and—"

"No, you didn't! I reminded you the doctor told us not to wax while using Retin-A."

Her reprove lit up the dark recesses of my mind—not in the RAM or cloud storage but in a removable external hard drive of my brain.

She had indeed told me.

The doctor had told me too.

And I'd forgotten.

Furthermore, I married a surfer and lived in fear he'd want me to join him in his beach endeavors. I stopped using it too soon, under the mistaken impression you can't use it and go into the sun for an extended time. It turns out you can do it with a high-SPF sunscreen without any problems. Retinoids cause new cell growth like a baby's new skin, so be careful.

Because I didn't use the product long enough, I didn't get the full results. I thought I'd have to choose between Retin-A and waxing, where waxing would definitely win. But now, with my current knowledge of use in the sun and my husband's nonexistent expectations of me joining him in the waves, I might give Retin-A another try.

Hormonal Blemishes

Blemishes seem to get you coming and going. I've not had this many zits since my teenage years. And hands down more now. When the hormones started going wonky, pimples started popping up. The ones that are deep under the skin and hurt like the dickens appeared along the jawline and hairline—a sure sign of hormone fluctuations. Like a boil under the skin, you can't do anything about them until they finally rise to the surface.

Oddly enough, my doctor recommended a nonprescription product you could only get from the pharmacist—Adult Acnomel. They had to order it because they didn't keep it in stock. Now, you can order it yourself online. It's a lightly tinted tube of wonder. I put it on at the first indication of ugliness starting, whether seen or unseen, and it's gone in no time. Not to mention, the tint helps to camouflage the blemish. Just keep an eye on the expiration date; they mean it.

Enlarged Pores

Whether clogged pores (zits) or enlarged pores, changes happen there too. There are two kinds of pores: the sweat glands and the oil-producing pores. The main causes of enlarged pores are excessively oily skin, decreased pore elasticity, and a clogged hair follicle. Dirt or makeup can block the pore, causing it to appear enlarged and develop a pimple.

Outside of an ongoing acne problem, enlarged pores are not a health concern. They are merely cosmetic concerns, and there are home remedies, like removing makeup and washing your face twice daily. Choose gel-based cleansers, avoid oil-based products, and wear sunscreen. Additionally, a better diet and increased water intake can help reduce enlarged pores, along with regular exercise to increase blood flow to the skin.[17]

Now, in my fifties, there are things I'll add to my regimen if they don't cost too much money or time. I have never been a night washer, and I took my makeup off in the morning until my mid-fifties when I started wearing foundation to cover the new age spots and the every-six-months precancerous skin freezing at the dermatologist.

I also lean on a product to minimize the appearance of enlarged pores around my nose and cheeks. Clinique has a pore minimizer I like called Pore Refining Solutions Instant Perfector. I use it only when I need a more finished look for headshot photos or special occasions. I used it a lot while dating Dean and for the wedding photos.

My former singles ministry pastor used to say, "Dating—the act of concealing; marriage—the act of revealing." Mark Lindsay hit the nail on the head.

Ticklishness

You could become much less ticklish with age. There are two kinds of ticklishness. Knismesis (**NIHZ**-meh-sis) is a light skin irritation, like a bug walking on your arm. You can tickle yourself in this way. Then there's the more intense laugh-provoking tickling, gargalesis (GAR-guh-LEE-sis), which stems from a person touching someone else in a sensitive area. You cannot tickle yourself in this manner.[18]

It's usually seen as a form of bonding between parents and children. As a child, I saw it as a form of torture. Still do. If Dean starts

Skin

to go for the sensitive areas, feet, or sides, I counter with, "Is that what we're doing now?"

Dean's CanDishItOutButCantTakeIt-itis kicks in, and he relents. "No, we are not. That window has closed."

I'm grateful I stopped to read his user manual. Regretfully, I have not yet cracked the code on my brother's user manual. Perhaps he's simply more committed to the sibling rivalry. After four-plus decades, there's still lots of tickling, poking, and "I'm telling" going on.

People view ticklers differently, and some people seem more sensitive to tickling than others. A lover's tickling can be welcomed, while a younger brother's could feel like torture. And sometimes, people relate tickling to an abusive relationship, so it's always a negative.

Tip: If you place your hand on top of the tickler's hand, your brain thinks you're the one doing the tickling and it's less effective.

While I've become less sensitive to the laughing (gargalesis) form of ticklishness, I have become much more sensitive to the irritation (knismesis) form—every loose hair down my shirt or bug flying by alerts my skin to a foreign object.

I'll write it off to a decade of lack of quality sleep.

This too shall pass.

CHAPTER 9

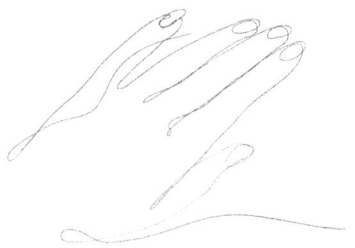

NAILS

Ingrown Toenails

Ingrown toenails are something my podiatrist said she'd seen more with teen boys over the years than any other age. She attributed it to them not wearing socks, shoes too small for their quickly growing feet, and general growing-boy uncleanliness. Then she admitted it skips right past the young adults' crowd and reappears in the over-forty group.

For more than ten years, ingrown toenails plagued me. Call it Murphy's Law or a lack of sleep, but I'd stubbed my toes more during this period than ever. The pain reverberated through my body and up to the stomach and head. In those moments, I didn't know if I'd toss my cookies or blackout. Bashing a toe is bad enough, but hitting an already red and throbbing digit made me question if I wouldn't be better off in a locked, padded room wearing a straitjacket. You can't stub a toe if you're doped to the hilt with Thorazine and drooling on yourself.

Partially out of frugality and scheduling and partially out of fear of fungal infections, I'd taken care of my own toenails all these years. Using my fingernail, I would pull the pestering big toenail out on top of the skin on the sides, but it wasn't a permanent solution. Frustrated with this new problem, I scheduled an appointment with my mother's nail technician. She instructed me to do exactly as I'd been doing. Then she added I should grow the nails longer to reach past the sides where they were digging in.

Sounded good, and it worked for a couple of years, until Hurricane Irma.

I waited for my brother to help fasten the storm shutters at the house, which I shared with my mother. I sent Joe a text inquiring about his impending arrival—no answer. As the hurricane approached, we hurried to protect the house. I started without him.

The house had a horizontal metal shutter system, a one-page general diagram, and a warped tutorial disc. I decided to wing it. How hard could it be? While Mom stress-baked inside, I carried each metal slab to the appropriate part of the house.

The neighbor saw me studying the diagram at a side window then came over and helped me slide each of the five shutters in place and tighten the bolts. One window down . . .

"Thanks for showing me what to do. My brother should be here soon to help me with the rest." I released him to finish his tasks.

"I'm almost done with our house. I'll help you until he gets here."

"Thanks!" I gladly accepted his generous offer. We'd completed all but the back porch in under an hour. I profusely thanked him and insisted he leave the rest for my brother, "who should be here . . . any . . . minute."

It turns out that two of Joe's friends had wrangled him to help with *their* hurricane prep. When he finally arrived, I had no energy left. The porch's sliding glass door shutters were installed vertically

Nails

with permanently attached brackets on top and bottom. Getting the vertical shutters in place can be tricky. I could barely hold the shutters while Joe nestled them onto their bolts.

When one of the slats stuck on the brackets, my brother kept saying, "Just get it into place."

Normally, we Floridians (the normal ones) weigh each action trying to avoid becoming a Florida Man headline news story: "Florida Man Caught on Camera Stealing Horses; Riding Them Home," "Florida Woman Attacked by Alligator after Falling in Canal," "Florida Man Caught Camping on Disney's Discovery Island, Says It Was 'Tropical Paradise'."

One year, I had the exact thought while stacking a crate on top of a patio table to reach the umbrella's folding pin. I envisioned the headline, "Florida Woman Injured Preparing for Hurricane." Naturally, I thought better of the circus-worthy feat during the hurricane season.

Not so this time. With the perfect storm of exhaustion, sweat dripping, and the irritation only a sibling can bring, I snapped and gave the metal slat a hard kick. Instantly, I regretted not wearing any of my three pairs of shoes and boots with steel toes sitting in my closet at the time (Skechers and Dr. Martens). Only once had I ever worn them for protection.

Instead, the foamy gardening shoes gave little cushion to the blow.

After some cursing (sorry, Joe!), blame-shifting (sorry again, Joe!), and some breath-catching, we finished the porch and endured the storm well, suffering no damage to the house and only a little to the yard.

At first, I thought I'd broken the toe—for the second time in five years. I didn't. I did, however, bruise it well, including under the nail.

Red polish helped camouflage the bruise as the nail grew out over the next year.

When a friend visited for a weekend, I mentioned touching up the red before we left for dinner. Jan offered to do it for me, and I relented when she assured me how much faster she'd be as a nail tech.

"I don't like the looks of this nail," she said.

"It's just the bruise growing out from the hurricane injury last year." I tried to read her face.

She pressed her lips together. "No. This is more than a bruise. I think it's a fungal infection."

My head spun. Jan did my third pedicure ever. In. My. Entire. Life.

With close relatives who'd fought the fungus for a decade or two, I'd purposely avoided nail salons because I didn't want to join the battle. Besides, I didn't trust myself to distinguish between clean and dirty salons.

"You can go to the beauty supply store and buy a topical. Give it three or four weeks, but don't mess around if it's not any better. Go see a doctor."

A month later, I tried to make an appointment with a podiatrist at the VA. Par for the course, they made me go to my primary care physician first. It took another two months to see the specialist. I had an appointment for early December.

The holidays are usually still sandals weather in Florida. Thankfully, I came prepared with flip-flops. She examined my toe and started cutting the nail. Before I knew it, she'd cut about two-thirds of the nail back on the big toe.

Without any pain.

"Most of your nail isn't attached." She nipped a little more.

Nails

The naked toe stared back at me. "Wow, there is no way to hide the nail now. I thought I'd have to make another appointment before you did anything more than an examination."

"I can finish today if you want."

"Please, I don't want to have to wait to come back again for this. And I don't want to spend the next two months stressing over it."

"I have two things I can do for it. We can remove the toenail and put you on a strong antifungal medication. You'll have to get a blood test about halfway through the nine-week course to ensure no kidney damage. I'll also give you a topical for a couple of weeks.

"Or I can give you the topical and send you on your way, but removing the nail and using the antifungal will give you the best chance at fighting this."

My heart sank. "I'll take the best-chance version." The extreme case. I knew I'd asked for pain, but better to nip it in the bud (accidental pun) than to circle this block again, possibly for decades.

She had the nurse get the numbing agent. The needle looked much larger than I expected; it hurt worse too. I had three pinholes by the time she finished numbing my big toe.

She put the needle back on the tray, and I leaned back to avoid watching the rest of the torture show. My head had already started wobbling and threatened to dislodge my stomach contents.

"Does this hurt?"

"No, just pressure."

She finished picking out dead skin and fungus, and then, with a numb, wrapped toe, I tread lightly in flip-flops back out to my vehicle with instructions for aftercare and a follow-up appointment for the next week.

The wrapped foot resembled something out of a cartoon, usually seen with dramatic throbbing and an antique car horn sound playing in the background (ah-oo-ga). I posted it on Facebook, and sympathy ensued.

Over the next two days, my toe hurt so badly that I borrowed my mother-in-law's unused walker—at ninety-one, she didn't use it—manufacturer's tags adorned it.

I managed comically. I couldn't put pressure on the wrapped area without the toe screaming. The gauze pulled from the base of the foot and other toes to the affected toe. Crutches would've made more sense, but you work with what you have. I asked Dean to get his office chair so I could use it as a makeshift wheelchair and glide easily to the bathroom from the living room, where I elevated the foot. During the night, I eased onto the floor and scooted to the bathroom with a modified crab walk.

The first night, in mid-scoot, he called out, "Where are you?"

"Down here. On the floor."

"What are you doing down there?"

After I debated how to answer, I decided to shelve the sarcasm for another day. "I had to go, and I can't walk. The chair won't roll on the bedroom carpet, so . . ."

At the end of the second full day, per the doctor's orders, I filled a plastic soaking bin with cool water and salt and removed the gauze. Most of it came off except where the nail once was. I cut it until a little remained and stuck my foot in the salinized water.

Every few minutes, I pulled at the remaining fibers dried in the nail bed. All but a few eventually came loose. Though I could finally walk without pain, I had big visions of the threads becoming one with my flesh, like something out of a horror movie. I went back to the doctor the next day without an appointment, hoping she'd have mercy and not make me wait until the next week's appointment. She obliged.

"The pain was so bad I couldn't get the rest of the gauze out. My husband couldn't stand the sight of the wounds, so he couldn't help. I just can't cause myself more pain."

She leaned over it with tweezers.

Nails

"Wait!" I urged. "Shouldn't we numb it again?" Yes, I knew I came across as a big baby.

Her face reflected the same thought. "I'll use a topical." She applied the gel and immediately leaned back in.

"Wait!" I implored again. "Doesn't it take time to numb?"

She tilted her head. "OK, we'll wait a minute." She passed the time asking me questions about my aftercare.

Letting her know how much trouble this whole endeavor had caused me helped me vent.

She rightfully ignored me and touched the nail bed with the tweezers. "How's that?"

"Better, no pain." I leaned back to avoid the ensuing nausea at the very site of the toe.

In less than a minute, she'd completed the task and put me on the road to recovery. Later, I read about a gel they could use with the gauze to avoid the issue I encountered. But the VA does not do luxury.

My next appointment went swimmingly, and the nail grew back remarkably fast. Six months into the process, it started hurting again, like an ingrown toenail.

And so it began. Again, I wondered why I always had to be the exception to the rule and the extreme of any case.

At a later appointment, she quickly nipped a spur of the nail. I returned to her office two months later, almost a year after she removed the nail.

She numbed the toe with numerous sticks from the needle. She removed just the outer edge of the toenail and applied acid to the root to keep it from growing up the outer edge.

So, no more ingrown toenails? On the contrary, I returned two months later with another spur at the base from the second removal. I found myself continually checking to see if it went sideways again. (Pun intended this time.)

Not long after, the nail grew back up the side, where she'd applied the acid. Unbelievable. It eventually grew back without giving me too much of a fit. I continued to monitor the nail and make sure it behaved.

 Tip: These things do not go away on their own. Check with your doctor if you suspect an infection or suffer from recurring ingrown toenails.

Hangnails

Another condition familiar to us as we age is hangnails where the harder skin at the base and edge of the fingernail seems to pull away from the nail. Aggravated with the drying conditions of winter, these jutting skin strips can cause pain and get infected if not dealt with properly.

Frequently washing your hands, submersing them in hot or cold water, or spending much time in a chlorinated pool can increase hangnails. Improper nail care and biting your nails can cause you to have them more frequently. Symptoms include redness, swelling, pain, and tenderness.

Avoid tearing the skin by biting or ripping. (My favorite method is the biting *while* ripping.) As with any open area of skin, it's more susceptible to infection. Wash your hands to avoid germs and bacteria. Use warm, soapy water, or apply oil or petroleum jelly and rub it in for about ten minutes. Use clean clippers or scissors to snip the hangnail. Cut only the exposed portion and then moisturize.[1]

To avoid getting a hangnail, keep your hands moisturized, wear gloves while working with your hands and washing dishes, don't cut your cuticles (seek a professional for help), don't bite your nails, and use a non-acetone nail polish remover.

Nails

 Tip: Try using a course emery board to carefully smooth down the rough parts without the risk of ripping open skin. Consider a cuticle oil if you're prone to hangnails.

Ridges

Ridges in the nails can form as we age too. Common and usually benign, the vertical ridges can be a sign of vitamin deficiencies or diabetes. Horizontal ridges can be a sign of a greater health condition. Mention these to your doctor right away. They can help with any conditions causing the fingernail ridges. Once the cause is gone, the ridges should grow out and disappear.[2]

CHAPTER 10

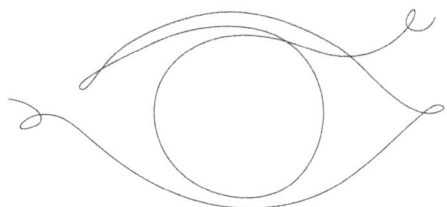

EYES

Glasses

Most everyone seems to endure vision changes. You're going along fine, and then one day, your arms are no longer long enough to see your phone's screen. The light is too dim in the restaurant to read the menu. The print is too small. It's subtle. If you haven't already worn glasses for most of your life, it seems corrective lenses are in your future.

You can use the drugstore cheaters (OTC readers) for only so long. Some of us stretch it out much longer than we should. Treat yourself to a proper vision exam and prescription, even if it's only for reading glasses. Having the right lenses can make a huge difference.

Most of us start seeing a change in our forties. I'd used the cheaters for a few years for reading books and menus, and they worked fine for most situations until we moved offices. I'd set my computer up with the monitor at an angle slightly to my left instead of the right to avoid direct glare from the window behind me. Nine months later, my right shoulder screamed. I finally caught myself leaning forward and to the left into the monitor to see the screen while leaving my right hand on the computer mouse. I'd done it so much that the repeated odd angle tweaked the right shoulder.

As the pain radiated in my shoulder, it dawned on me that I needed to see my optometrist. (Only I would get my eyes checked for a shoulder injury.) She said the cheaters would only get me so far since they are only one strength, and I needed two: one for reading papers and one for reading my computer screen. I heeded her advice and treated myself to progressive lenses. Unlike bifocals, with their distinct line of magnification, the progressive lenses allowed for three distances and melded seamlessly. In my glasses, the top has no prescription, so I can drive with them without slipping my glasses to the end of my nose to look over them. The middle is for the computer monitor, about two feet away. The bottom portion is for closer reading.

In their frames store, I cautiously chose the single accessory I'd wear with everything. Every day, like picking out one pair of shoes to go with all your outfits. I get one purse to go with everything until it rots off my arm, but I don't have to wear a purse on my face. I sprang for the works, including blue-light blocking tint. The budget doesn't stretch for expensive shoes or purses. I made the exception for the glasses but refused to spend $695 again on a second pair just for wardrobe accessory choices.

It took about two weeks to get used to them and not feel nauseated, but I adapted. My brain made my eyes find the right spot on their own. Because of the seamless merging between all three distances, anything from near to far was in focus.

Since I'm careful with glasses and because my prescription hadn't changed, it was several years before I needed a new prescription. The doctor said I had two different conditions that worked against each other, which kept my eyes stable—until the sixth year.

Eyes

I'd known for months the time had come. New glasses. And the pressure of once again choosing the perfect frames.

The doctor said I could use a stronger prescription, one eye more than the other. She also pointed out I still had 20/20 vision but just needed a little help. I asked about contacts, which she'd mentioned the year before. I marveled with reservation at how the eyes could adjust to progressive contacts.

She'd said, "The brain just figures it out."

With an appointment to try contacts and my prescription in hand, I went to their store to peruse the vast selection of frames once again.

From a countertop sign at a department store in the 1990s, I learned that I should wear rectangular frames. After stopping only for those, I narrowed it down to three.

"Did you find something you like?" an attendant asked.

"I suppose these might do, but I like mine a whole lot better," I whined.

"You can use your frames, but if they break, you'll have to buy new frames and then pay for new lenses." She looked through my file on her computer. "It looks like they're six years old. I'm not trying to sell new frames to you, but I'm a little surprised they haven't broken already."

I sighed.

"Let me try something." She took my glasses to the back to check their inventory while I held my breath. "We don't have them here, and they don't make them anymore." As my heart sank, she added, "But I can order them from the stock our supplier still has on hand."

Finally, some good news.

The next week at a birthday dinner, when I mentioned to my family my vision remained 20/20, but the doctor told me I needed a new prescription, they chided me.

The doubt set in.

Fear of my optometrist being a charlatan grew. I turned to the internet and found that it's true and not just the ravings of a mad eye doctor. Having 20/20 vision means you can see clearly at a distance of twenty feet away—not necessarily perfect vision. Your optometrist might not be able to get you seeing perfectly, but it's usually much better than without corrective lenses.[1]

A screenshot of the article summary proved my case. I shared it with the family. Boom. Mic drop.

My glasses came in mere days before the COVID-19 shutdowns hit the news. A week later, they called to reschedule my contact fitting appointment for May. They said they were closing for the entire month of April.

After a few moments, I fiddled with the new glasses when panic set in. I called back and ran down for another frame adjustment. I don't know why I wouldn't have said something sooner, but over the previous six years, the old frames made indentions on my head above my ears.

When I asked her to avoid the current ruts behind my ears, she raised an eyebrow as if she'd also wondered why in the world I hadn't said something sooner. Years sooner. She made a few more adjustments, and we achieved success. "It may still take quite a while for the indentions to disappear."

Though I was too old for my 1980s hairdo, I'd hoped the era's shaved hairstyles didn't make a comeback until the grooves disappeared.

Contacts (or Teaching Old Dogs New Tricks)

The eye appointments for contacts did not occur in May as scheduled but in June of 2020, according to COVID-19 state guidelines. I arrived to a mask mandate and temperature gun to

Eyes

my head. Too hot. I had to sit in the corner until I cooled off from the hot Florida car ride. It reminded me of a trip to China in 2003 with SARS (COVID-19 precursor) in full bloom. My host missionary family told me about their recent trip home, where the dad popped hot at the Guangdong airport. They let him grab a cold soda and hold the can against his head for a minute. He then passed the temperature gun test. I question safety measures at home and abroad.

Once upstairs and in the examination chair for my fitting course, the technician gave me the eye chart exam. "Is one better, or two? What about three, or four? Better or worse?"

The mask pushed my breath upward and into my eyes, drying them out and complicating the difficult determining of minute differences between slides. We managed after repeated requests like, "Wait, go back. Do those two again."

She then managed to get the lenses on my eyeballs with all my flinching. In my defense, there is a lot of unintentional blinking and twitching involved when someone tries to stick something in your eye.

Then the doctor came in, looked through my file, and ran me through a few more eye chart questions. She then asked me to get my phone and read something.

I whipped it from my purse and read a few lines from a Facebook post. *Looks like I'm having a good-eyes day,* I thought to myself.

"OK, let's go to the contacts room where you can try to put them on yourself. Afterward, you can go to the front desk, and they'll arrange a follow-up appointment for next Friday."

"Is that when I'll get the prescription contacts?"

"No, you're wearing them now. We'll recheck your eyes and make sure the prescription is correct. Plus, you'll have time to adjust to putting them in and taking them out. You'll still have to wear glasses for small or up-close actions like threading a needle, but these should get you through most scenarios."

Until then, I'd thought each lens had multiple distances from top to bottom, like my glasses. Wrong again. Each lens had a different prescription: left eye for closer reading, right eye for farther out.

It all happened so quickly. "But I thought I needed training contacts without a prescription to practice with."

"Nope. You're wearing them. Follow me." She then led me to the contacts room and sat me at one of three tables. The technician gave me a case to put the lenses in until I could get them back in my eyes.

After many attempts and frustration, I asked, "Got any tips for me?"

"See if you can come from the backside of your head and hold the upper eyelid with the nondominant hand. Then hold the contact on your dominant hand's index finger, while you use the middle finger of your dominant hand to pull down the lower lid, and seat the lens."

Sounds easy if you say it fast.

Yes, it worked better than my willy-nilly haphazard way.

"You did good!"

After about twenty minutes, I said, "I'd hate to see someone doing it poorly."

"Men. They don't adjust well. I think we women can do it better because a lot of us are already used to poking around our eyes with makeup." She wasn't wrong.

Though I improved, I felt I could still use more insight. Dr. Google had tutorials with more advice. There is a fabulous video, "Contact Lenses for Beginners," from Dr. Joseph Allen on Doctor Eye Health's YouTube channel.[2] He said to make sure you didn't have them inside out, as I'm sure I did twice the following week.

Eyes

It felt like I had something else in my eye, like a loose lash or piece of sand—it is Florida, after all. The first time, I chased a phantom all day but never took the contact out until I got home, then just assumed the foreign debris came out with it. (Remember, I'm not very good at paying attention sometimes.) The second time, I drove home and went straight for the bathroom. Once I removed the contact, the debris sensation stopped. This time, I noticed and played with the contact. Sure enough, I'd put it in inside out.

Dr. Allen discussed how you could tell by shape—if it's correct, the lens will be a tighter U-shape and a looser U if inside out (more like a suction cup than a bell curve). But honestly, it looks so similar to me both ways. Then he said another way to tell is "the taco test." The lens will stick to itself when it's sitting the right way.

My reading vision improved, but I'd lost most of my distance vision (ahem, I never had a problem with distance before). I could see fine to drive, but reading signs proved difficult. I couldn't read a license plate unless the automobile stopped right in front of me at a red light.

As it turned out, I needed the follow-up appointment for fine-tuning. The following Friday, she did a quick eye chart exam and adjusted my right eye a bit more for distance and my left eye a bit more for reading. My eyes weren't too bad anyhow, so the difference between the two wasn't stark, and the brain adjusted.

She gave me enough for the weekend and said they'd have more Monday. When I called on Monday and asked if they were in: nope. Tuesday? Nope. Wednesday, I called again, and they said they should hear from the manufacturer by Monday. More COVID-19 delays. The contacts finally came in, and I had enough for my second trial period. They informed me that "buying in bulk gets the price way down."

"Well, sign me up for a year's supply." The price fell to less than fifty dollars per month. For normal eyes, the price is far less, but I

Hot Mess Express

had to buy ones for presbyopia ("a visual condition which becomes apparent especially in middle age and in which loss of elasticity of the lens of the eye causes defective accommodation and inability to focus sharply for near vision"[3]). Naturally, I needed the more expensive lenses.

Contacts are a better choice for workdays, where my glasses were on so much for computer and paper reading that I started getting dents and spider veins on the bridge of my nose due to the heavier frames. On days not at work, I opted for the glasses and eventually tossed the lenses as soon as I returned home from work as I only needed them for the occasional recipe, mail, or bedtime reading. I also opted for the glasses during crafts to see the fine details better. I couldn't even see the date on my watch or thread a needle.

After the first time in the pool with contacts, I didn't wear them on swim days. It's too much of a hassle to remember to keep my eyes closed every time I go underwater or jump in. I play in the water like a child, acknowledging the judges before each dive and practicing my aquatic ballet to the alternative music of the eighties or Dean's reggae. (I find sunning on a floaty boring.)

Sometimes, I forgot to remove the contacts and wore my glasses wondering why I couldn't see the television.

The contacts "shine" when I'm exhausted, when it's hard to see anything through the lenses because of glare or blur. I'd squeeze my eyes shut and open them, and I could then see clearly for a second or two, sometimes enough to get the job done, sometimes not. In those cases, I tossed them and settled for the glasses. I found this unacceptable and kept my eye out for lightweight glasses frames I liked so I could ditch the contacts altogether. Being a thrifty person, I kept using the contacts until only a handful remained for occasions when I wanted to see without glasses. When they're gone, they're gone.

Eyes

Cataracts

The glowing halo around lights at night? My optometrist said it's the beginning of cataracts. She said most people will get cataracts as they age if they live long enough. Discouraging.

They can make reading or driving at night more difficult. It builds slowly, but eventually, cataracts can obscure your vision. They leave your eyes cloudy to see through and cloudy in appearance too. Besides the halos, symptoms can also include worsening night vision, sensitivity to light and glare, and a more frequent need for glasses and contacts prescription changes. See your doctor if you notice these changes or any on the complete list below.

- Clouded, blurred or dim vision.
- Trouble seeing at night.
- Sensitivity to light and glare.
- Need for brighter light for reading and other activities.
- Seeing "halos" around lights.
- Frequent changes in eyeglass or contact lens prescription.
- Fading or yellowing of colors.
- Double vision in one eye.[4]

Cataract surgery has become much more prevalent in America. The principle of supply and demand made this procedure more affordable, but most insurance companies don't consider it a necessary treatment. LASIK surgery will only take about fifteen minutes and will cost you anywhere from $3,000 to $5,000. Of course, risks are involved, and you could still need reading glasses afterward.

Depth Perception

Depth perception can decrease with age. Cataracts, glaucoma, and refractive errors—the regular reason most of us need glasses—can all lead to depth perception problems, but an exam can rule out age-related issues. People who wear bifocals or trifocals in glasses are more susceptible.[5]

Patients who undergo LASIK surgery to correct nearsightedness, farsightedness, and astigmatism can also experience better depth perception.[6]

For years now, I've hit my shoulders on doorjambs as I passed through; I thought it might be caused by lack of deep sleep for many years combined with my extra-wide shoulders. Now and then, someone pokes me to check for shoulder pads, which I never needed, even in the eighties. But now the problem may be the newly developing cataracts my doctor mentioned at my last checkup.

It's too soon for me to consider LASIK. When I do, I can improve my clarity and depth perception. In the meantime, I'll stick with glasses.

Thinning Eyelids

As a child, I'd laughed at my father telling us, "I'm heading to the bedroom to check my eyelids for pinholes." A nap.

Seemingly thinning eyelids have made me feel like I have actual pinholes.

A South Korean study showed no signs of age affecting skin thickness on the eyelids, but something happened.[7] I became convinced when a friend mentioned having to use a sleep mask after she'd turned sixty. More than a decade younger than her, I'd been trying to find the right sleep mask for two years.

In my teens and twenties, I could sleep until noon. Daylight, clock lights, and television light never bothered me then. Even shift work in the army and the Kennedy Space Center demanding daytime sleep never bothered me with the light flooding in.

Why now?

The sleep issue lay at the top of the suspect list. Again.

Eyes

As previously discussed in chapter 4, "Insomnia," changes in hormones wreak havoc, and ambient light can affect your sleep even more. If, like me, you already have problems achieving the deeper levels of sleep, the slightest interruptions bring you out of sleep completely. Anything you can do to eliminate the extra light and sounds will help you achieve a deeper sleep and stay asleep longer.

Adenosine, a chemical found in your cells, builds in your brain throughout the day and then informs your body when to sleep. In addition, your circadian rhythm plays off of natural and blue light from your television, computer, and smartphone. It is a major component of your body's internal clock for sleep and wake times. When light floods in, your body suppresses chemicals, including the sleep chemical melatonin.[8]

In the darkness, your body releases melatonin and your circadian rhythm thinks it's time for bed. It makes us feel sleepy and continues to release to lull us into deeper sleep cycles.

Exposure to light around bedtime can delay melatonin by about ninety minutes, which can make the difference between a good night and a bad night of sleep.[9]

The simple sleep mask to the rescue. There are many sleep masks on the market to help keep out light. I'd tried a freebie with a pillow order and purchased a handful online and locally. I received one for Christmas with extra room for your eyes so you wouldn't smudge your makeup. Great for back sleepers, but not for this side sleeper. Too lumpy.

Too bad.

My favorite mask is from an inexpensive three-pack I got online. I gave one to Dean for when I'm up before dawn for work and have to turn the lights on. It leaves room for the nose without letting in light and has an adjustable strap for the right tension. On the weekends, I slip it on just before dawn, during one of the many times I wake. Tinted stickers darken the alarm clock's light, so I don't need the mask until then.

Droopy Eyelids

Droopy eyelids can make putting on makeup a challenge. For years, I'd worn a modified smoky style of eyeshadow with a dark shadow on the lid, slightly winging out, and a lighter shadow toward the brow. Then, in my early fifties, I kept finding a white streak in the crease where I missed the dark shadow.

A crevice.

A fold.

So frustrating. And it's just starting. (Cue the violins!)

Diabetes can be an underlying issue that causes the whole eyelid to droop (ptosis). If a disease is not causing muscle weakness and droopy eyelids, you can have surgery for the eyelids interfering with sight or for cosmetic concerns.

If only the skin is sagging (*blepharochalasis*), like with my eyelids losing their elasticity, surgery is also an option, but insurance most likely won't pay for either surgery unless the sagging interferes with sight.[10]

 Tip: Metallic eye shadows build up in the cracks, accentuating the lines. Stick to flat or matte eyeshadows, especially near crow's feet. Also, adjust your application to have a light color on the lid and brow line with a darker color in the crease.

CHAPTER 11

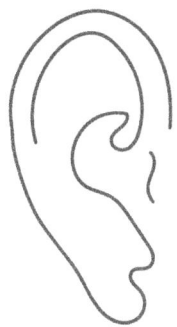

INNER EAR

Motion Sickness

A forty-minute line for a roller coaster? No problem. I'd waited longer in many lines. In my teens, I rode the Loch Ness Monster at Busch Gardens repeatedly with a season pass. I'd done the Hulk coaster at Islands of Adventure ten times consecutively. But the last time I went to the fun park, I waited with my brother at a restaurant table while the younger ones and my sister went to ride the coaster. The dizzying effects of motion sickness are too great for me now. They have been since my early forties.

It's an inner ear problem, specifically the deterioration of the hair follicles and other hearing mechanisms as a cause of ringing in the ear (tinnitus), equilibrium issues affecting balance, and overall hearing loss. Sometimes words become indistinguishable or hard to hear with ambient noises.[1]

Sometimes wax buildup can be the cause, but if it's age-related, hearing aids can help with the natural aging process. Check with your doctor before everyone gets tired of hearing you ask, "What?" Believe me, I will. I know plenty of people over the age of seventy. One can't hear half of what we say but refuses to admit the problem is his. The rest of us must be mumbling.

Roller coasters cause great dizziness now, and the pressure on an airplane flight gets worse each time too. The motion of takeoffs and landings makes it almost not worth flying anymore. A trip is not fun when you're constantly eyeing the paper bag in the seatback in front of you. Dean and I now decide on trips based on the length of a car drive.

Some of the symptoms of motion sickness are dizziness, nausea, and vomiting. Other symptoms can include belching, headache, and sweating. Hyperventilation can be found in some extreme cases.[2]

Pointers to help manage motion sickness comprise picking a middle seat on a boat or plane and sitting forward-facing on a train, pretreating with ginger, and curbing your food and drink intake before and during travel. Visit your doctor to talk about your choices.

10 Tips to Beat Motion Sickness[3]

1. Take control of the situation. Be the driver not the passenger; keep your eyes on the horizon; distract yourself with conversation; avoid reading.
2. Curb you consumption. Limit food and drinks before and during travel.
3. Get into position. Choose the middle of the plane near the wing; pick lower, center levels on a ship.
4. Equalize your sensory cues. For seasickness, lie down; sit facing forward on a train.
5. Talk yourself down. Use positive speech about yourself and the upcoming experience; breathing techniques can help too.

Inner Ear

6. Get desensitized. Read a book for five minutes, then put the book down; repeat this cycle a few times, then increase the time to ten minutes, etc.
7. Pretreat with ginger. Two grams of ginger thirty minutes before travel can help. (Check for interactions with blood thinning medications.)
8. Get in touch with your pressure points. Try wearing pressure point devices.
9. Ride it out. Your body adjusts on the seas after three days.
10. When all else fails, medicate. Dramamine or Meclizine help for severe motion sickness, or try the scopolamine patch available on most cruises.

Tip: I recommend always having a balcony room on a cruise. It provides a much-needed respite from the crowds and can be a haven if the boat breaks down or you get quarantined to your room.

Vertigo

As I previously mentioned in chapter 4, "Insomnia," I've had issues with loose crystals in the inner ear, which can also make you dizzy. It's called benign paroxysmal positional vertigo (BPPV), which people over age sixty are more likely to get. It's also the easiest type of vertigo to treat.[4]

The sensation happens when a crystal rides your natural wax past the hair follicles. The sensation stops when your head is still.

My doctor did the Epley Maneuver. This is one of four main maneuvers, each resembling the actions required of a wooden labyrinth game, where you try to get the metal ball into the proper hole by tilting the box to guide the ball. Likewise, the loose crystal is directed back into the proper part of the inner ear.

> **Tip:** Before attempting to treat this problem yourself, see your doctor. It's important to know what kind of vertigo you have and which ear it's affecting before trying any remedies.

You can try medication to help alleviate the symptoms, but it can take a while to go away on its own, and with vertigo, time is a luxury you cannot afford. (Unless you have a life of leisure and a personal driver, which most of us do not have.)

Menopause can lead to dry itchy ears, ringing in the ears (tinnitus), or hearing loss or oversensitivity among other changes. For any ear concerns, ask your doctor about home remedies or diet changes. Keep a food diary to show during your next exam.[5]

Ear mucus can wax and wane with age (pun intended, thank you). I never suffered from dry ears, but frequently awoke to goopy ears. Doctors oppose cotton swabs used to remove excessive wax. The old saying goes "never put anything smaller than your elbow into your ear." Check with your doctor for causes and safe ways to equalize the amount of ear wax.[6]

CHAPTER 12

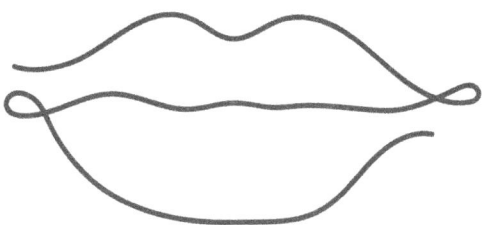

MOUTH

Halitosis

Halitosis is bad breath by any other name. Good dental hygiene takes care of most of the causes of bad breath. It includes flossing daily, brushing twice daily, and using a gum stimulator—a rubber-tipped metal stick my dental hygienist introduced me to. I called it a torture device as I kept slipping with it and jabbing my gums, testing the limits of my salvation (just kidding, there aren't any). I later teased her that her name became a cuss word.

After I adjusted to it, I asked if I could stop using it at my next regular six-month checkup. She said, "Why would you stop using something if it works?" Her name has been mumbled a time or two since.

Good dental hygiene can help prevent heart disease and help you keep friends.

You run into the occasional bad breath from something you've eaten like onions or coffee. But then there's the entirely different kind of bad breath, chronic halitosis.

Hot Mess Express

We had a sweet older lady who sat behind us in church—fifty is older when you're thirty. She had problems getting around. From what, I do not know. Amazingly, I didn't ask—my mother would be proud. After church, when we all rose to leave or mingle, she made her way to her feet with the help of her husband and leaned in for a hug. She exuded love. But her breath!

Several middle-aged to older people with chronic halitosis crossed my path over the years. It's not food, such as garlic, or even cigarettes. Bad breath is not pleasant.

Oral malodor is not something you want to be around.

Stank-mouth strains relationships.

My nose is extra sensitive, and since one fateful flight home from Germany during my army years, I've had barometric pressure headaches—similar to migraines but not nearly as debilitating. Since then, I'd become smell sensitive. I skirt the perfume counters at department stores and can't tolerate most men's colognes either. With my super sniffer, imagine my surprise when I tasted my own bad breath. I cupped my hand over my mouth and exhaled. Disgusting.

I'd brushed and flossed regularly, used my torturous gum stimulator, and stuck to a six-month cleaning regimen. I've even used a tongue scraper on occasion. Panic rose with my heartbeat. Not me!

Naturally, I turned to Dr. Google. (A word of caution about using "Dr. Google": a webpage cannot diagnose you or give you a clean bill of health. All you can do is gather information. That information should be used cautiously and should never replace a trip to your doctor.) Having ruled out dental issues, I explored the sinus cavity as a cause. Sinus infections or bacteria in your nose and sinus cavities can cause offensive odors. A saline nasal wash can help relieve this condition.[1]

Besides dental and diet causes, another cause could be stomach issues like acid reflux. I have dealt with a lot more in recent years and recently bought the larger bottles of antacids, but my dentist hasn't mentioned the eroding of tooth enamel—a sure sign of a bigger reflux issue.

I bought a battery-operated sinus cleanser. I also purchased nasal sinus drops from TheraBreath. They make several products for various mouth and sinus causes of bad breath, from tonsil stones (bacteria collection on the tonsils) to dry mouth, which can be from medication or smoking.

The bulky battery-operated sinus cleanser proved hard to use. You had to fill the water tank, then place the proprietary saline pod over the tank and press down the top, which engages the unit. The pods cost a lot, more so when you clamp down on them before you add the water to the tank. I've had to toss a perfectly good pod more than once because once you lift the chamber, you need a new pod to reengage the system. In addition, you have only one shot at the flow button. If you let up, you'll need another saline pod to start the unit again. My hands have always been weak, but this button pushes the limits of my hand strength as well as concentration.

Perfectly lining up the nasal rubber tips wasn't the easiest task either. Then, you have to hold the not-so-light unit level and press the flow button for the forty-five seconds it takes to run the saline water mix through your sinus cavity. (Closer to two minutes if you don't hold it steady and level. It can feel like an eternity as you lean over the sink to catch the leak if you can't get a tight nasal seal.) But, hey, maybe you're more coordinated than I am.

My ear, nose, and throat (ENT) doctor told me about an inexpensive method I should've stuck with after my deviated septum surgery: ear bulb and cheap saline packets—a box of a hundred for less than ten dollars, compared to forty bucks for ninety proprietary saline packets.

Oh, neti pot, why did I forsake you? Sometimes, simple is best.

Hot Mess Express

After implementing the saline rinse at nighttime, I still noticed the particular bad taste on occasion. The TheraBreath nasal sinus drops did the trick each time.

Bad breath felt more like a warning sign of aging than the gray hairs in my thirties. As a side note, nothing I've mentioned in this book besides the IBS is anything I ever had to deal with as a "young" person.

When looking for an effective mouthwash that won't kill your mitochondria (makes energy for your cells) or affect your microbiome (overall bacteria network throughout your body, which helps absorb nutrients), as a regular mouthwash can, look for a product without harmful ingredients such as alcohol, chlorine dioxide, chlorhexidine, cocamidopropyl betaine, poloxamer 407, formaldehyde, or saccharin.[2] A number of products fit that bill, such as Tom's of Maine Natural Mouthwash, Aesop Mouthwash, Oral Essentials Lumineux, Georganics Oil Pulling Mouthwash, Auromere Ayurvedic Mouthwash, The Natural Dentist Healthy Gums Antigingivitis Rinse, and JĀSÖN Healthy Mouth. You could also make your own with distilled water, baking soda, and sea salt.[3]

Dr. Nathan Bryan suggested eliminating regular mouthwash as it kills good bacteria too. You need these to process certain vitamins and minerals, which help you stave off high blood pressure and other ailments. He mentioned that two-thirds of American adults use mouthwash regularly, which corresponds to the fact that two-thirds also have high blood pressure. He further suggested foregoing the fluoride toothpaste and rinse at the dentist's office. And lay off the antacids for the same reasons. We're shutting down nitric oxide production and killing the bacteria that help us fight hypertension and other vascular dysfunctions, like type 2 diabetes, dementia, and Alzheimer's. We are trading a stomach ache for a headache and ruining our microbiome (how it's all connected through the cardiovascular system).[4]

Tip: Instead of popping an antacid, try ginger, peppermint, yogurt, or apple cider vinegar. Protect your nitric oxide.[5]

Yellowing Teeth

The parade of changes continues with yellowing teeth. I've seen commercials with young, beautiful people talking about their yellowing teeth and how to get them white. Aside from extreme dental issues, it doesn't seem that too many young people need to whiten their teeth. Me in my late forties? It's a different story.

 Tip: Lipsticks with warm tones can make teeth look yellow. Cool tones can make them look whiter.

Taking it to heart, I implemented the tip above and tossed my reddish-brown lipstick, even though it looked great with my "fall" coloring. I found a pinkish-red color to replace it. Eventually, the new cool color wasn't enough, and I asked my dental hygienist if I should try the whitening service they offered. She told me my teeth weren't bad enough to pay two hundred dollars to get whiter. She recommended the OTC home version from Crest for fifteen dollars.

Happily, I saved the cash.

She said, "Years of coffee, tea, and dark juices can leave stains. OTC products have become very affordable."

Later, I got a multiuse paste and blue light mouthpiece kit, as they use at the dental office, on a deal-of-the-day special for less than forty dollars. An OTC whitening toothpaste buys time between whitening kit sessions.

Tooth Sensitivity

From time to time, I also now suffer from a little tooth sensitivity. When it first rears its ugly head, I switch to Sensodyne Pronamel; in no time, I'm back to regular paste—without fluoride. Try it and ask your dentist about the sensitivity on your next visit.

Canker Sores

Canker sores (aphthous ulcers) can be stress-induced, but I can't always pin them on stress when they appear. And truthfully, I bite the inside of my mouth regularly, which can form a traumatic ulcer, feeling the same. Jamming a toothbrush into your gums can cause a traumatic ulcer too. (Yep, assaulting my mouth with toothbrushes and gum stimulators . . . it's what I do.) I blamed canker sores in the bitten and jabbed areas instead of my lack of learning how to eat. After five decades, I still can't seem to learn how to properly chew food without chewing my tongue or inner cheek.

There's a lack of evidence for any true cause of canker sores. But it's thought stress and certain acidic foods can bring them on. Canker sores are more prevalent in teens and young adults, usually during stressful times. They also appear more around the time of a woman's menstrual period. And you're more likely to get them if a parent gets them.[6] Since it's a younger woman's problem, why mention it?

Thank you for asking. I believe the hormonal change triggers them. I didn't have them as a younger gal, yet I had plenty of stress. And plenty of hormones. My mother shared with me how she had a stress-induced bout with canker sores in her forties. They clustered and ran down her throat—a particularly nasty attack, indeed.

Settle down, Dean, my slightly germophobic husband; they are not transferable—unlike cold sores, which are on the outside of the mouth, usually the lips, and are a part of the herpes family, with

Mouth

up to 67 percent of the world population suffering from them. No, we, the 20 percent of the population suffering from canker sores, can't pass them on. Thankfully. But having a canker sore can make us more susceptible to catching something else, like Herpes Simplex Virus-1, the lip cold sore, because the canker sore is an open wound.

Choking

Choking on my saliva is another feat I'm perfecting. How many decades will it take for me to learn how to swallow my spit correctly? Not just saliva, but also coffee, water . . . it could be any drink. At one of our after-church lunches, Dean's ninety-two-year-old mother choked on her drink.

Wrong pipe.

So familiar.

She prevailed, but now I can't stop thinking about how much worse it's gotten for me in the past five years—let alone how much worse it could get in the next forty.

Coughing while choking is good. It's a sign your body is correcting the problem. It's all good until the coughing (and breathing) stops, then it's time to intercede. Look up the Heimlich Maneuver and learn it.

 Tip: If you find yourself alone when you choke, dial 911 and run to a neighbor you know is home or out near traffic to flag someone down. Don't wait to start moving. Some areas have implemented texting to 911. Make a plan now and practice.

People over sixty-five years of age are several times more likely to choke on food than young, preschool-aged children. Doctors blame this condition (dysphagia) on the weakening of the muscles, compounded by the choice of soft foods over foods requiring chewing.

> **Performing the Heimlich Maneuver on Yourself**[7]
> 1. Call 911.
> 2. Place your fist slightly above your navel.
> 3. Grasp your fist with the other hand.
> 4. Bend over a hard surface for leverage (table, chair, countertop, or railing).
> 5. Thrust your fist inward and upward.

Fewer and weaker muscles compound swallow issues as we age.[8]

Reduced saliva from conditions like dry mouth, acid reflux, diverticulosis, and other disorders can contribute to choking, which can damage the esophagus or cause pneumonia.[9]

Wrong pipe.

But when the cause of choking is plain old aging, there is something you can do. At-home exercises, such as the ones below, can strengthen your tongue, or a speech-language pathologist might have you do other activities to improve your range of motion and various swallowing techniques.

Tongue-Strengthening Exercises

- Stick out your tongue as far as you can. Put something flat like a spoon or tongue depressor on your tongue. Push against your tongue with the flat object, and push your tongue against the object. Hold for a couple of seconds. Repeat 5 times.
- Repeat the exercise above 5 times. This time, put the spoon or depressor below your tongue instead.
- Extend your tongue as far as possible to the corner of your mouth while pushing against a depressor. Hold for a couple of seconds. Relax. Repeat on the other side of your mouth. Repeat the whole process 5 times.
- Extend your tongue to the bumpy part on the top of your mouth right behind your teeth. Then curl your tongue back

Mouth

toward the back of your mouth as far as possible. Hold for a few seconds. Repeat 5 times.[10]

Other Movements a Speech-Language Pathologist Might Have You Do

- Inhale and hold your breath very tightly. Bear down like you are having a bowel movement. Keep holding your breath and bearing down as you swallow. This is called a super-supraglottic swallow. Repeat a few times.
- Pretend to gargle while holding your tongue back as far as possible. Repeat.
- Pretend to yawn while holding your tongue back as far as possible. Repeat.
- Do a dry swallow, squeezing all of your swallowing muscles as tightly as you can. Imagine swallowing a vitamin whole, without water. Repeat a few times.[11]

I'm sunk again because if I put anything on my tongue, it might activate my very sensitive gag reflex. Pretend to gargle. Do I pretend to gag too?

These exercises would most likely be done in conjunction with other types of swallowing exercises that target other areas of the mouth and throat, such as cheek- and lip-strengthening exercises. Your doctor will help you narrow down a regimen specific to your swallowing issue. Do them in order so you don't forget to do them all.

Not sure it's going to help me since I set out each night to brush, floss, and poke all in the same order, upper outside to inside, bottom, and left to right. But I sometimes can't remember if I've already done one section or another. I then complicate the matter by choosing the next day's clothes while I do my oral hygiene tasks. It's like driving and hoping you had all green lights since you can't remember traveling the past section of the road.

Hot Mess Express

Swallowing pills is slowly getting worse too. I've never been good at taking medicine or vitamins, gagging them back up half the time. Then I saw a video of a guy explaining how to do it more easily. He said to put one or all of the pills in your mouth and work them to the back of the tongue. Take the glass of water and imagine the water going over the tongue and collecting the pills like a river would then swallow when it hits the back of the throat.

Since I grew up in the seventies with *Land of the Lost* on our television every Saturday morning, I picture Mr. Marshall, Will, and Holly in their yellow expedition raft going down the great underground waterfall and into the lost land of dinosaurs and Cha-Ka. It does help to picture something that's best for you in order to mentally symbolize the pills going down and not coming back up.

 Tip: Take a sip first to wet your dry mouth, and don't let the pills sit long on your tongue or they will stick. Do it all quickly.

CHAPTER 13

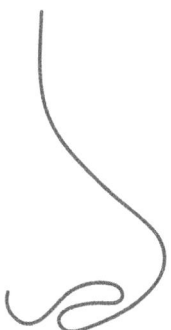

NOSE

Snoring

Snoring can create stress in a relationship. When I first married Dean, I enjoyed peaceful nights, except for the hormonal lack of deep and REM sleep—and the animals. He had two cats, and I added my one dog to the mix. Two months later, due to various ailments, only one cat remained: Tucker. Even though cats are nocturnal, the nights were mostly peaceful, even with my insufficient sleep.

Four months into marital bliss, snoring entered our lives, and I became accustomed to the midnight shuffle to the guest bedroom.

Snoring is the vibrating sound of air flowing past relaxed throat tissues during breathing. Nearly everyone will snore at some point, but it can become an ongoing issue for some. It can indicate a serious problem and be problematic for everyone else in the home.[1]

Causes can be anything from how your mouth and sinuses are formed, including a deviated septum, to alcohol consumption, allergies, and other causes of nasal congestion. Even your sleep position and weight gain can cause snoring. A narrowed airway causes the airflow to become more forceful, increasing vibrations and the sound of snoring.[2]

Sleep Apnea

As discussed in chapter 4, "Insomnia," sleep apnea is a major source of insomnia. The associated breathing pauses are also the main culprit for snoring, as the person snorts themselves back into a regular breathing pattern. If you snore accompanied by any of the following, it is recommended that you see your doctor:

- Witnessed breathing pauses during sleep
- Excessive daytime sleepiness
- Difficulty concentrating
- Morning headaches
- Sore throat upon awakening
- Restless sleep
- Gasping or choking at night
- High blood pressure
- Chest pain at night
- Snoring is so loud it's disrupting your partner's sleep[3]

Men are more likely to snore, but women do it too. Dean said if I fell asleep on my back, I could snore for up to an hour. Even though I thoughtfully presented him with a video containing audio recordings of his snoring, he failed to produce any proof of my disturbances.

Nevertheless, I took him at his word. I hated to interrupt his snore-fest, so I tried to hit the back position first, then shift to my side before drifting off to another wonderful night of broken sleep. It seemed to do the trick.

He had an appointment for his problem, for which I suspected allergies. The doctor had no clear conclusions yet offered surgery.

Nose

"Did you tell her your snoring is intermittent, and sometimes you go weeks before it rears its ugly head again?"

Visibly angry when the seven-hundred-dollar bill arrived, with most of the costs due to the surgical fee, he waved the paper. "Surgery? She only ran a lighted scope up my nose for ten seconds."

After a neighbor said they'd struggled with snoring until they discovered a certain allergy spray, I purchased a store brand of it. It took some coaxing of Dean, who doesn't like taking medication. We joked about the name, depending on where we got it, which was Plonaze from Publix or Walnaze from Walmart. Later, I stumbled across the Sam's Club six-pack for a fraction of the price. (No, it's not Samnaze; we just call it nose spray.) It worked so well that I've rarely seen the guest bed since. They should rename it "Better Than Surgery Allergy Spray."

My snoring has not yet gotten to the point of interrupting his night, and with no indications of snoring during my previous sleep study, we aren't too worried about it. However, some of the side effects of a snoring issue can be serious, so it's nothing to dismiss. If you suspect you have a snoring problem, please see your doctor, as these can be some of the complications:

- Daytime sleepiness
- Frequent frustration or anger
- Difficulty concentrating
- A greater risk of high blood pressure, heart conditions, and stroke
- An increased risk of motor vehicle accidents due to lack of sleep[4]

Though the symptoms and complications listed are for the person snoring, many of these complications can be experienced by their beloved sleeping in the same bed because of their interrupted sleep.

Deviated Septum

A deviated septum is a condition that either you're born with or occurs due to facial injury or trauma. The bone and cartilage divider between nasal cavities can become crooked, causing breathing difficulties. Most people have some misalignment, but only extreme cases need attention. See your doctor if you have any of the following symptoms:

- Sinus infections
- Nosebleeds
- Facial pain
- Headache
- Postnasal drip
- Loud breathing and snoring during sleep
- Obstruction of one or both nostrils
- Awareness of the nasal cycle
- Preference for sleeping on a particular side[5]

Though I'd suffered headaches, nosebleeds, and frequent stuffiness for as long as I could remember, I don't know if my deviated septum existed at birth or if roughhousing caused it. My ENT suggested surgery to repair the deviation. In 2007, I gave him the green light. He performed a septoplasty to correct the septum.

A friend had it done three times. Each time, it returned to the deviated position.

Spoiler Alert: Mine did too.

Pain permeated for about five days. I couldn't leave my face alone for two minutes, often forgetting the tenderness. I saw cartoon birds dancing around my head with each touch.

Gauze packed my nostrils, feeling like pool noodles crammed in there. I flinched when the doctor reached to take the gauze out on the fifth day.

"Don't you trust me?" Dr. P. frowned.

Nose

"You don't understand the pain each time I zing myself."

"It will be OK."

He gently reached up with his small fingers and eased the gauze out.

No pain.

Only freedom.

Air flowed in. For the first time in a long time (maybe ever) I could jog and still breathe through my nose—a real game-changer. In the army, they had yelled at me for breathing through my mouth while running. The cold air through my mouth would hurt my throat during the freezing German winters. But I couldn't get enough air otherwise. It changed after surgery. The constant stuffiness disappeared too.

However, the freedom lasted for only four months when I clogged up again.

The procedure could have been repeated as my one friend did, but I also had another friend who had the procedure done and had to go back in to get it cauterized to stop the bleeding. Because of their experiences and mine, I chose to leave it alone.

When I stuff up at bedtime, I use a method I stumbled across a couple of years ago on the internet. It's time-consuming, but it works and beats getting out of bed again. It's great if you're opposed to taking drugs. Apply pressure with your thumb between the frontal sinuses (between your eyebrows). Press lightly for two seconds, then release for a second; repeat for up to two minutes. I find it usually clears within thirty seconds.

There's a sweet spot for it around the part of the brow as it curves into the nose. It might take a few seconds to find, but you'll know when you have it as you push and release it. Press in this area off-center to the right or left to clear the corresponding side of the nose.

I suspect a sagging face may also play a part. We had a surveyor at my bookkeeping job who said women aged like the Nazis melting at the end of *Raiders of the Lost Ark* whereas men get more character. Rude? Yes, but I think he's onto something for people in general, not just for women. Gravity's effects are real, and I can see my face melting like a figure in a burning wax museum. When I'm slightly stuffy as I lie down in bed, I can smush that same part over the bridge of the nose toward the forehead, and I can breathe again; let go, and I'm clogged again. I'm sure there is surgery for that, but I'm not desperate enough yet. Like winter, a facelift is coming, especially if it'll clear the sinuses—bonus. I'll put it on my wish list for my sixtieth birthday.

Sinus Infection

Sinus infections can increase with age too. The nose continues to grow and change as can symptoms of postnasal drip, runny nose, and dryness. These increase as we age. Reduced hydration can result in thicker mucus. The reduced ability to blow effectively can leave mucus behind, increasing chances of infection, especially in postmenopausal women.[6]

Rinsing the sinus cavity with a bulb, neti pot, or another device, as discussed in chapter 12, "Mouth," can help release mucus. Be sure you use clean water (distilled or boiled) with a salt or saline mix to avoid further infection.

 Tip: Some doctors suggest that regular or daily sinus rinsing can increase infections and to only do it when an infection is present, not daily.[7]

Migraines

Though my headaches are sinus-related and often brought on by weather or strong scents, many women suffer from hormone-related migraines. Women can suffer from migraines at a rate of three times as much as men, but they should decrease as you pass from perimenopause into menopause. Hanging in there can be difficult. Along with pain, usually on one side of the head, you can have flashing lights, nausea, light sensitivity, and vomiting.[8]

Migraines can be brought on by

- bright lights
- foods or drinks
- hunger
- lack of sleep
- stress
- strong scents[9]

Dropping estrogen levels are believed to be a cause for women right before their period. With the fluctuation of estrogen during perimenopause, women can experience an increase in migraines. If they've experienced migraines for a long while, menopause may bring relief. If migraines plague you, keep a food diary to see if you can identify any trigger foods. Eat meals at regular times. Go to sleep and rise at the same time each day (yes, even on the weekends—at least within an hour of normal times). Finally, relax with deep breathing, exercise, and massage.[10]

As with anything mentioned in this book, there are treatments, even for migraines. See your doctor and bring a log with you. Try to crack the code before you get there, or you could be sent away to document your habits and then return later to discuss. Your doctor can help with frequency and pain.

CHAPTER 14

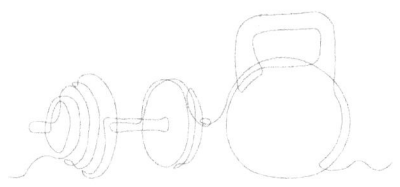

MUSCLE TONE

Muscle Tone

My mother grew up in California with her mother, while her grandparents remained in Kansas. Still very young when they passed away, she has few memories of them. She told me about seeing her grandma, Sadie Simpson, in her Salvation Army uniform. Another favorite recollection is sitting in her large lap and playing with the fat on her upper arm. Batting it back and forth.

It's doubtful women today would be so vulnerable, even with grandchildren.

The old rule I mentioned in chapter 8, "Skin," about how women over fifty shouldn't wear sleeves above the elbow comes to mind. Maybe it's Florida or the heat, but women don't seem to adhere to that rule anymore. With women now proudly revealing what our mothers would have hidden, you look like a prude when you sport three-quarter-length sleeves.

Since I've joined the ranks of the over-fifty crowd, I struggle with the rule as I pick through the sales racks. My arms are still fairly firm, and I can still make an impressive bicep muscle, but there is presently less muscle tone overall. I haven't seen the gun show in the mirror in years, never mind muscle strength. My three-sets-of-thirty-sit-ups gymnastics days are in the rearview mirror. The days of the popular high school girl pointing at my six-pack abs during gym period change-out and making sounds like "eww" are also behind me. The only thing left from those days is the counseling I have yet to receive.

In her podcast, *The Storyteller's Mission,* Zena Dell Lowe discussed in episode 12 how to make your characters credible and believable. To explain this topic, she used the example of the movie *Entrapment* with Sean Connery and Catherine Zeta-Jones. He's the thief; she's the insurance investigator setting him up. Zena pointed out the absurd notion of an almost seventy-year-old doing feats of acrobatics almost too much for a young man in his prime. True. She made the point that they'd not shown him continuing to work out to explain how he could pull it off at an age when most men retire.

As a former gymnast, I can attest to that fact. After not working out during one summer, I found even the basic movements more difficult, even as a tiny fourteen-year-old.

There is a reason we don't see octogenarians in the Olympics alongside the young competitors. As we age, our physical abilities diminish. Our bodies change. We simply can't do at sixty, fifty, or forty, what we once did at twenty.

We over-fifties aren't supposed to do sit-ups anymore. A modified abdominal exercise routine is recommended, and it doesn't include crunches either. Instead, modified core exercises like chair planks, seated knee lifts, and oblique side bends are suggested to avoid back injuries.[1]

Sit-ups are hard on your back because they work your hip flexor muscles, which run up the thighs and around to the lower

Muscle Tone

back and can pull on the back. Sometimes a backache is caused by your hip flexors in the front.[2]

Having suffered from back pain since my army days, exercising is on again / off again. (Lately, it's more related to problems from chapter 9, "Nails.") Even during my time in the army, they were already modifying the jumping jack with the "side straddle hop." The army phased out the sit-up by the end of 2020 and made room for more useful fitness tasks closely related to soldiers' combat readiness, like deadlifts, power throws, and drag-and-carry moves.[3]

Resistance isn't quite as futile as a Star Trek movie would have you believe.

You can build strength, muscle mass, and flexibility with resistance bands or by using your body weight, making normal household tasks easier, like carrying grocery bags and climbing stairs. Flexibility exercises can help you move well and avoid injury as you age.[4]

Tip: Squat exercises, with or without weights, will increase your thigh mass. Proceed with caution, but the results will outweigh any concerns about mass increase. If you are able, do it!

I'm transitioning into a better exercise routine.

And a better wardrobe.

The days of wearing a twentysomething wardrobe are behind me, but I don't want to dress like I've given up. Dean admitted he thought the yards of fabric I wore when we met added ten years to my appearance! So, I've been transitioning the wardrobe to be more age-appropriate while trying to remain stylish and comfortable.

One of my favorites is still the stretch jeans, a modern marvel. Goodbye to jeweled back pockets; hello to fabric g-i-v-e—a muffin top reducer—and the return of blood circulation. When these jeans are pulled up, a lot of body mass rises with them and then resettles—much lower than it used to be, but higher than without them now.

When I put them on, I have to jump in place to get everything to settle where I want it.

Cellulite

Regardless, life's better with stretch jeans, but I've noticed they are not all created equal. A white pair I own seems to accentuate the cellulite, the dimpling in the flesh, seemingly accumulated with every year and pound—donation pile candidate.

One of the longtime married men at the office said, "Jeans really hide a lot." He stared off . . . probably back to 1974 when his wife could get away with short-shorts.

Regrets, I have a few. Not fully taking advantage of my youthful body is one. I've always been a bit body-shy. (Understandable after the locker room incident.) Twins from my gymnastics team had cellulite at the tender age of thirteen. But I didn't notice it in myself until my thirties.

Cellulite is more common in females than males, due to the different distributions of fat, muscle, and connective tissue. Most women may experience cellulite at some point in their lives, though the cause is unknown. Contributing factors may include dropping estrogen levels and slowing blood flow. And the aging skin sagging increases cellulite development.[5]

Other factors mentioned were genetics, diet, and lifestyle activity. Too much fat, carbohydrates, and salt with too little fiber can contribute to cellulite. Other factors are smoking, lack of exercise, and general sedentary lifestyles.[6]

Muscle Tone

Most of those got checked off on my list. With this in mind, I set out to see if I could reduce the appearance of my cellulite, starting with dietary changes. My research included three methods.

Food Combining—an oddly named method because it's about separating foods. You're supposed to eat your protein twenty minutes after the carbohydrates. This theory suggests meat takes longer to digest and backs up your carbs to let your body absorb more sugars. I saw no impact and only did it based on a recommendation from a friend, though there's no evidence that food combining diets improve digestion or enhance weight loss.[7]

Vegan—eliminated all meats and dairy products but allowed cream for my one cup of decaf coffee. This might have been further impeded by my mother supplementing my diet with carbs to help fill me. My mother lost eight pounds, which I found on my thighs. This also reinforced the thought that not all calories are the same. Carbs were friendlier to my mother than they were to me.

No or Low Carbohydrates—by greatly reducing my carb intake of bread, desserts, chips, and so on, this dietary change made a difference in my cellulite. The fat cells were reduced with the overall weight loss of twenty pounds. It changed the appearance of the amount of cellulite. If you choose this method or similar, like Keto, there are apps to help you track your food and help you balance the fiber, protein, and carbs.

There are medications in creams applied to the skin, like caffeine to burn fat and retinol to thicken skin, and several other treatments to reduce the amount of cellulite or reduce its appearance, like the following:

- Acoustic wave therapy
- Laser treatment
- Subcision
- Vacuum-assisted precise tissue release

- Carboxytherapy
- Endermologie
- Ionithermie cellulite reduction treatment
- Radiotherapy
- Laser-assisted liposuction
- Ultrasonic liposculpting[8]

It doesn't appear that any have scientific results.

> Alternative or supplemental therapies include caffeine, grape seed extract, or ginkgo biloba. These agents have been applied topically, orally, and by injection, but none of them have proven effective.
> Some people wear compression garments to reduce the appearance of cellulite. These garments try to compress arteries and increase blood and lymph flow to reduce visible cellulite.[9]

Then came Dr. Berg. He suggested new science pointing to three problems causing the appearance of cellulite: atrophy, circulation, and collagen bands dissolving. I'll spare you the details and, instead, point you to what he says are the solutions. For muscle atrophy, increase muscle tone by stimulating the glutes, thighs, and hips with lunges, squats, retro walking (a methodical backward walking, outdoors or carefully on a treadmill), and sprinting (try ten-second bursts, two or three times to start, but only if you're healthy).[10]

For the circulation problem, he suggested rebound exercises (like jumping on a trampoline) and infrared light therapy, which increases melatonin, antioxidants, and sleep. A dry brush or massage on the area could also help increase blood flow. Finally, to help the collagen band, you could try fasting intermittently for twelve or more hours between meals or prolonged fasting. You could also try an aromatase inhibitor topical cream (such as DIM—a concentrated cruciferous version).[11]

Muscle Tone

If you decide to try any of the exercises, first, start slowly. Overdoing it is counterproductive. You want to be able to do the exercises with the correct form—sloppy won't get you where you want to be. Second, if you're sore, don't keep going; wait to recover. Third, create enough stimulus for the muscle. You want to "feel the burn" then let it heal. Fourth, get enough sleep or you won't have the energy to complete the exercises. Also, your insulin and cortisol levels will be too high and will counteract your efforts. Finally, give it enough time. It could take up to eighteen months to see the full results.[12]

For strength training, begin with a comfortable weight with which you are able to do twelve to fifteen repetitions in correct form but ending in muscle fatigue. You have to take the reps to muscle fatigue in order to build muscle. After you start slowly, you will begin to feel results like being able to do more weights or go farther before exhaustion. This is not going to the point of injury or pain. If you join a gym, they will usually have someone who is trained and can walk you through this process. Or join a local strength-training class.[13]

When you become comfortable in your new routine, you will decide whether to go with more weights and fewer repetitions for more muscle or less weight and more reps for muscle endurance. For each rep set, no matter which method, you are looking to get to muscle fatigue, where you just cannot do one more rep in correct form but quickly recover to do the next set in only a few minutes. You can start with one to build muscle then switch to the other to maintain and build endurance.[14]

 Tip: Take progress pictures in order to see the improvement and to motivate you not to give up.[15]

Hot Mess Express

This is a natural segue to the shaper garments, but they can make your pants sit unnaturally if the garment is too tight. A too-tight garment doesn't let the pants' seams rest somewhat recessed into the, um, where the good Lord split ya. We've all seen the women wearing the support hose, and everything is flush with the cheeks with no natural crack depression. You can tell she's getting help.

The point of it all is to keep your cheating secrets to yourself—remember the feminine mystique. Shaping garments and support hose are better with skirts and dresses.

Another great secret is the slip shorts. They are an awesome substitution for dress slips of yore unless you're trying to keep the light from shining through the material. Once I discovered the shorts, my slips were either donated or trashed when the elastic died. I kept one for the light-blocking scenario. The slip shorts will act in the same way as the traditional slip, hiding panty lines and muting loud panty colors, but not completely; choose your undergarments carefully.

These little secret keepers also allow for clothing to flow naturally. Without the concern of panty lines, the slip shorts and shaping garments give you confidence and discretion. They give you the confidence of a little girl on the recess playground with shorts on under her dress. You can once again hang upside-down from the monkey bars. Just don't hurt yourself.

 Tip: Liposuction and dieting do not remove cellulite. But, reducing fat intake will decrease the amount of fat pushed through the connective tissues. A balanced diet and exercise may reduce the appearance of cellulite.[16]

Muscle Tone

Exercise isn't enough by itself. For me, it'll be low fat, low carbs, high protein, along with age-appropriate lean muscle-building exercises.

My plumber passed away in someone's backyard while fixing a pipe. He worked out five days a week for hours at a time. No fifty-year-old looked buffer, but he ate fast food each day for lunch. Probably dinner, too, as a bachelor. He couldn't out-exercise his bad diet and neither can we.

Diet isn't enough by itself, either.

You will be as bad off as my plumber with a sedentary lifestyle. You might have great arteries, but your muscles and bones will fail you later in life.

Eat right for clean insides. Exercise for a strong outside. And stretch so you don't get a hitch in your giddyup.

I suspect you can live a long life by simply eating well. It's all well and good if you have someone to carry you around for the last twenty years of your life. Exercising is very important to stave off the immobilization you can see set in with so many seniors.

But with a healthy diet, I suspect even if you did not exercise but instead stretched regularly, you'd win the race of the tortoise and the hare.

Sometimes genetics can bless or curse you, but most of us have to make choices.

"Habits we form now will last a lifetime." I've heard it so many times in my life, but it's strange because, for the life of me, I can't remember who said it. (Did I mention my sleep issue?)

Not everybody will develop an exercise routine. If you do, great—fantastic! But if you don't, remember to eat better and stretch.

Stretching has to be done regularly to keep muscles long and flexible to avoid falls and injuries.[17] You can even stretch out the sciatic nerve pain in some cases.

> **Tip:** A quick online search will yield a treasure trove of exercise and stretching routines. Don't wait until your condition is so bad that you need cortisone shots, surgery, or biweekly visits to the chiropractor.

The iliotibial (IT) band can also cause difficulties. Like the hip flexors, it can manifest in lower back pain. Stretching can relieve the IT band. At one point, the pain interfered with my already poor sleep. I'd woken numerous times with one hip screaming, only to wake up another half-hour later with the other side on fire. As a side sleeper, those were my two choices.

A massage therapist mentioned the IT band, and my chiropractor also mentioned it. They both put their thumb right on it, and I flinched big time. When Dean rubbed it months earlier, I assumed the cellulite and connective tissue caused the pain. I just thought it stemmed from my being a delicate flower. (Press the canned laughter button here!) But when two people mentioned the IT band in less than a month, I listened. I found a video online with some stretches, which brought some relief until I could get to physical therapy for some individualized instruction and guidance.

At my physical therapy appointment, she guided me through some stretching exercises for the IT band and hip flexors. She gave me flyers with notes we'd made and emailed videos of the stretches for me to look at later when I'd already forgotten all of her instructions. Perfect.

Apparently, when I felt better, I stopped stretching. Two years later, I had problems sleeping on my side. I kept waking up around 3:00 or 4:00 a.m. with my hips screaming, which further hampered the sleep issue as a side sleeper. Again, my chiropractor mentioned the IT band. I'd completely forgotten about the previous bout until

Muscle Tone

I got a book contract and started editing this chapter. Note to self: keep stretching.

There's a reason the experts freak out when professional athletes injure themselves. I've heard it said many times: once you injure yourself, it weakens the muscle or ligament, and you're likely to reinjure the same area.

If muscle aches, pains, strains, and pulls are the question, then diet, exercise, and stretching are the answer. They're not a fix-all. They won't bring back your lost youth—your smooth skin, tight muscles, and dimple-less skin. This body won't last forever, but I'm just trying to make it to the finish line with grace and independence. Longevity.

Sagging

Once gravity takes hold, you know you're on the downhill slide. Besides cellulite, the other main areas I've noticed are my sagging breasts and derriere. Like I said, with the jeans, it's all riding a little lower and jigglier back there. And up front, well, I didn't used to be able to hold a pencil under my boobs. Over the years, I've had a number of master bathrooms with the toilet across from the sink mirror. So, you can see yourself while you . . . go? Sometimes, I'd gotten naked for a bath or shower, then stopped to go before jumping in. A little self-conscious while sitting in front of the mirror, I'd put my long hair in front to cover my breasts, like a mermaid. Now my hair is long again, but it doesn't cover my breasts anymore. Depressing. If that isn't bad enough, it took me far too long to figure out the cause of my ruined game of mermaid—gravity.

After forty, the doctors like to schedule annual breast exams and mammograms. A friend used to say, "They're turning your teacups into saucers!" I have lumpy, dense breasts, so it's a bit more painful. The technicians have to handle the breasts much more now after fifty to get them into the perfect position.

I've donated or returned so many items now because I misjudged gravity's effect on my body, including certain strapless bras without the underwire support system. I tried two different sticky/self-adhesive reusable bras, but they are no good unless you're a youthful size-A cup. I purchased a couple of strapless dresses with the elastic tube top to wear around the house after the pool or after work. Not my best look, so they went back.

Strapless swimsuits? Not anymore.

Tube tops? Nope. They're as bad as the dress. I thought the weight of the extra material from the dress made it hang badly. No, 'twas the sagging of my boobs that made my boobs look so saggy. Even with a strapless bra with underwire, they lacked altitude.

 Tip: Avoid strapless dresses and tops unless you are more flat-chested, as most clothes do fit better with smaller breasts. The grass is always greener.

Only one of my strapless bras continues to muster the job. It's from Le Mystère. I call it the Iron Maiden. You'll pay good money for it, but it's worth it. To ensure the correct size, go to a higher-end department store offering fitting services.

Speaking of bras fitting you properly, there's the Breasts-in-the-Middle Test—"when your . . . bra cup apex should be halfway between the top of your shoulder and your elbow. If lower than this, your band is probably too large and not giving your breasts enough support." (I'd always blamed the strap.) For a D cup or larger, you may need a bra with seams in the cups for more support.[18]

During perimenopause, your breasts and nipples can sometimes become sore or tender, like during the menstrual cycle, except

Muscle Tone

this can last for days, weeks, or months. Because they left my ovaries when removing my uterus, I still had cyclical, PMS-like symptoms, such as breast tenderness for a couple of days here and there. Painful enough at times I'd have to warn Dean not to touch them. One time, the pain lasted for more than two months.

Just as I started to freak out, I consulted Dr. Google, who assured me sometimes it's the diet.

> **Dietary Steps to Minimize Sore Breasts**[19]
> - Eliminate caffeine
> - Eat a low-fat diet
> - Reduce salt intake
> - Avoid smoking
> - Take an over-the-counter pain reliever
> - Ask your doctor if switching birth control pills or hormone replacement therapy medications may help

Fluctuating hormones can also affect breast tissue making it more sensitive. The part that reassured me is that soreness is not usually associated with breast cancer. This new pain can be associated with hormone replacement therapy.[20] Consult your doctor for any of the following:

- Thickening or lump in your breast or under the arm
- Pitting of the skin, giving it an orange peel look
- Nipple discharge
- Nipple retraction (turning inward)
- Swelling, redness
- Change in size or shape of your breast[21]

Even though my body is relatively new to Dean, he likes to tease me about my losing battle with gravity. While I ignore him, he'll take a hand under one breast and raise it just a tad then act like it fell several inches. Dramatically, his hand wobbles with big movements, then settles into small aftershocks, often lasting a few seconds, longer when I'm not wearing a bra. My straight face gives way to laughter every time.

However, his CanDishItOutButCantTakeIt-itis acts up when I do it to his chin, stomach, or . . . other parts. Good times.

Bladder

The bladder is another weakening muscle. Oops, tinkles when you laugh? Some of you went through it when your pregnancy put extra pressure on the full bladder. Well, here it comes again. Here are some changes that can occur to your bladder as you age:

- The bladder wall changes. The elastic tissue becomes stiffer and the bladder becomes less stretchy. The bladder cannot hold as much urine as before.
- The bladder muscles weaken.
- The urethra can become partially or totally blocked. In women, this can be due to weakened muscles that cause the bladder or vagina to fall out of position (prolapse).[22]

Your bladder might not hold as much urine as before, and that can be annoying, but you'll want to seek medical help if you notice any of the following:

- Signs of a urinary tract infection, including fever or chills, burning when urinating, nausea and vomiting, extreme tiredness, or flank pain
- Very dark urine or fresh blood in the urine
- Trouble urinating
- Urinating more often than usual (polyuria)
- Sudden need to urinate (urinary urgency)

My maternal grandmother constantly struggled with urinary tract infections (UTIs). Symptoms may consist of fever, chills, and burning when urinating. Natural cures include drinking plenty of

Muscle Tone

water, vitamin C, and cranberry juice. Urinating more frequently and after sex reduces the risks of UTIs, as do avoiding spermicides and wiping from front to back.[23] If these haven't worked or if you have a prolonged or high fever, seek medical help.

At least we ladies don't have to worry about prostate issues complicating the matter. We have our own issues affecting the bladder, like certain medications or medical issues, but the next time you sneeze, cough, or laugh and pee just a little, consider exercising the muscle.

Kegel exercises strengthen the bladder muscles. The individual contractions of a Kegel workout require you to squeeze the pelvic floor muscles just as you would if you were trying to stop urine flow.

Kegel Exercises[24]

- Contract the pelvic floor muscles and hold for a count of 3.
- Relax the muscles completely for a count of 3.
- Repeat 10 times and work your way up to one set of 10 to 15 squeezes three times a day.

A friend of mine swears Kegel exercises saved her from a much too early future of urine pads and adult diapers at the tender age of sixty. The Premarin (vaginal estrogen cream) my doctor ordered for vaginal dryness also helped my occasional bladder leak issue by applying the remaining bit of cream left on the applicator to my urethra each night. (Reminder: the urethra is where your urine comes out. You're welcome; I saved you from searching the web and seeing what cannot be unseen.)

Leg Cramps

Leg cramps can strike during the day or in the middle of the night. Reduction in your body's ability to make more estrogen can bring on these spasms. Reports of muscle cramps increase as we age—one-third over sixty and a half over eighty years of age.[25] In our youth, the primary cause is dehydration and exertion. But as the body ages, the estrogen receptors all over our bodies deplete, increasing joint and muscular pain.[26]

When the pain rouses you from sweet slumber, if you are fortunate enough to achieve deep sleep, you have several ways to address the cramps, including:

- NSAIDs (non-steroidal anti-inflammatory drugs)
- Pickle juice
- Vitamin B-12 supplements
- Magnesium and calcium supplements
- Natural muscle relaxers like chamomile tea
- Natural anti-inflammatory substances like turmeric[27]

A study done by a neurobiologist hypothesized and blamed an "overstimulation of motor neurons serving the muscles." They thought introducing a strong sensory input, like acids or strong spices, could block the motor output causing the cramps. The study resulted in such success that they started a company selling a drink made from ginger, cinnamon, and capsicum. Their study supported the old wives' tale of drinking pickle juice to alleviate cramps.[28]

Your doctor can prescribe muscle relaxers if stretching through the cramps or the natural remedies don't work for you.

Restless Legs Syndrome

For some, Restless Legs Syndrome (RLS) is the cause of leg cramps. Associated sensations within the limbs are described as "crawling, creeping, pulling, throbbing, aching, itching, and electric," which ease with movement. The uncontrollable nighttime twitching and kicking, sometimes associated with a condition called

Muscle Tone

"periodic limb movement of sleep," can interrupt sleep, affecting your day and quality of life. Talk to your doctor if you think you might have RLS. They can test and treat conditions that often accompany RLS, such as peripheral neuropathy, iron deficiency, kidney failure, or spinal cord conditions.[29]

CHAPTER 15

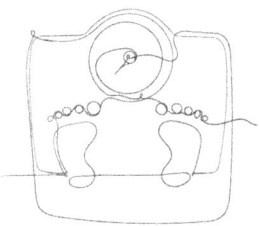

METABOLISM AND WEIGHT GAIN

One evening in my mid-thirties, we crowded around the stove at a friend's house. She lived with her much older parents, who had a physician's scale in their kitchen. While waiting for our weekly show to start, we dished out dinner. Before my turn, I stepped onto the floating black plate of the scale.

I knew the answer already: 115 to 118 pounds. Tapping at the bottom weight to nudge it to the right, it seated into the one-hundred mark. The top weight, pushed all the way to the left at zero, moved easily past the ten-pound mark. With no divot to rest in, like the bottom weight, I scooched it little by little. Tap, tap, tap until the scale balanced.

My face flushed while writing this—similar to back then. Breathing became shallow and quick as the inevitable caught up with me. Well, not quite at that moment. Denial kicked in, along with some champion-level blame-shifting.

"Your scale's off," I said defiantly.

My friend calmly replied, "No, it's not."

Her mother added, "The doctor came here yesterday and calibrated it. Whatever you're reading is right."

Lightheaded, I stepped down in disbelief. My mind swam with all my eating escapades. More than once, I'd eaten a pound of bacon in one sitting. I'd eaten more Sloppy Joes than any of the guys during a high school Super Bowl party, including the football team members. I'd polished off a regular-sized bag of chips with a can of French onion dip in one sitting at least once a week during my army years. Did it all catch up? Finally?

"Why? How much does it say?" she asked.

Not sure who asked, I turned to face both. "One hundred twenty-eight."

Confusion clouded their faces. "What did you expect it to be?" They asked in unison.

"Ten pounds less."

They held their composure, but their chubby faces lovingly welcomed me to the club.

"I thought my jeans shrank in the wash. Apparently, I'm just not a size three anymore."

Laughter abounded from the duo. My friend mumbled, "I don't think I've been a size three since fifth grade."

My weight had always been deceptive. Throughout my life, I'd weighed more than others of my size. A lot more.

"I'm really dense," I explained once to my family.

"Yes, we've always known that about you," they teased about my mental acuteness.

"My mother had me tested," I replied when teased.

Because I was still tiny enough at a year old for my mother to bathe me in the kitchen sink, the doctor recommended testing to see if I also had intellectual disability in addition to the slow physical growth. Tests showed normal cognitive function.

Metabolism and Weight Gain

But ten pounds on my petite frame is comparable to twenty or thirty on average-sized folks. As they say, if only I could go back to when I first thought I was fat—back to when my clothes hung loosely off my petite frame.

Muffin Top

Britney Spears made the super low-rise jeans popular in 2001, while the term "muffin top" entered our vocabulary in 2003.[1]

With the midsection bulge exacerbated by the low-waist pants, I think we all now know what to call the roll of fat over the top of the jeans. Some of us from personal experience. (My hand is raised.) The discovery of my love handles came around the same time as the scale incident. It's when I started paying attention to the changes.

Though my 5′2″ stature would have you believe I shop in the petite clothing section, I do not, as my legs account for a disproportionate amount of my height and got me into the army without a waiver for height. As I had a disproportionately short midsection, the super low-rise jeans fit me nicely without too much risk of anyone mistaking me for a plumber.

Nevertheless, I sat in my chair at work one day in the early 2000s, staring at my boxy computer screen. With hands-on-hips to stretch my back, I marveled at this new addition of body mass. It didn't even strike me as weight gain but simply a mysterious addition.

Admittedly, my genetics blessed me with a great metabolism. Combined with my physical activities, it prolonged my girlish figure for many years. Until it didn't. I'd never struggled with weight issues, so when the careless eating caught up with me, I felt like a millionaire gone broke. I harkened back to a colorful phrase I grew up hearing from my father about looking up the word *sympathy* in the dictionary.

Before that, I could eat whatever I wanted, as much as I wanted. Now I look at ice cream and gain five pounds.

My current scale (which I inherited with the marriage) is a real jokester. To turn it on, press the plate with your foot, wait for it to zero out, and then step on with both feet. In a quick moment, my tale is told, for good or for bad. But this scale likes to mock me. At the last minute, it jumps up a half-pound, never down. I can hear it say, "Take that with you!" and wink at me.

That stupid scale gets me every time.

As I mentioned in chapter 14, "Muscle Tone," stretch jeans are your friend, but perhaps they're more of an enemy. We don't notice the changes as quickly as in traditional jeans, which would have us lying flat on the bed trying to close the button and zipper far before the stretch jeans' waist digs in.

As I also pointed out in that chapter, the shaper garment is a lifesaver. In addition to the numerous benefits already stated, you can wear your favorite full-coverage cotton underwear without worrying about panty lines. (I ditched the silky underwear decades ago when I moved to Florida and became acquainted with real humidity—it creates a condition called Swamp Butt.)

Thickening Thighs

When the Florida wind gets blustery and threatens to reveal my not-so-sexy cotton undies or I need the effect of a slip under my material to make the dress or skirt flow naturally, I wear a certain pair of slip shorts. They also keep my thickening thighs from rubbing together when I'm twentysomething pounds up in weight.

If I'm a skinny girl, why are my thighs rubbing? Well, obviously, I'm no longer the little girl my parents used to tease had knots tied in her legs to have knees. I've often said being single for so long is a disadvantage. I could quote scripture about the blessings of being

Metabolism and Weight Gain

married and having children, but the truth is getting married young is the blessing of ignorance. Marrying young helps you mature. Moreover, having children helps you grow up. Since I waited until fifty to marry and have no children, I'm only as mature as the given situation dictates, and I see my eighteen-year-old self in the mirror.

Time stood still for three decades.

Then reality came crashing in and conflicted with the status quo. My mind had problems reconciling the changes in the body. I think we all do to some degree, but women like me don't have pregnancies and childbearing to blame it on. Much to my mother's dismay, babies didn't cause my paunch.

My pants got tighter in the waist, butt, and thighs. My tall winter boots got tighter as I gained weight in the calves. With increased thigh mass, I crossed my legs with more difficulty. In addition, my shirts got tighter in the chest. My bras and underwear became tighter too.

Though I now admit some of the middle-aged spread is to be expected, I swore I would not buy a "fat" wardrobe. I encourage you to be comfortable in your clothes, but not at the expense of losing the ability to notice when you pack on extra pounds. Stay within a small range of a couple of sizes. And unless you live in Hawaii, do not buy a muumuu.

Clothing brands now vary to the point where you have to try everything on. I fit well into a lower size number and the next size up, too, depending on the designer.

As a reminder, it's not the number on the tag that counts but your overall health. When I start overflowing my bras, underwear, and waistbands, it's time to rethink my habits.

Slowing Metabolism

A slowing metabolism makes women feel like they have to starve themselves to see a downward trend on the scale, while men seem to have a passing thought about weight loss and lose ten pounds—not fair, but it is reality. "Men generally have more lean muscle mass, and men's bodies burn through visceral fat reserves more quickly."[2] They use more energy for activity instead of saving it for later.

Visceral is the gut or organ fat. A doctor once told me if you lie down on your back and the fat falls to the sides, then it's just regular surface fat. On the flip side, if it stays perched like a beach ball, that's the visceral (organ) fat and very harmful. Mostly, you see it on men, but some women carry it too.

More muscle equates to a faster metabolism and a leaner body. Weight lifting will help recover lost muscle mass due to the lower hormone levels associated with aging. An appropriate workout can help you reenergize your metabolism or keep you from losing muscle in the first place.[3]

The metabolic process is a chemical reaction in all organisms, but metabolism is simply how your body transforms food into energy.[4]

The good news is you don't have to be a bodybuilder to make it happen, but you need weights, resistance bands, or your own body's weight to get the job done.

Cardio will help younger people, but for the over-forty women, we don't get the same benefits. We need to walk ten thousand steps (give or take) each day, do resistance training using bands or weights to gain back lost lean muscle, and do high-intensity interval training (HIIT) to help increase metabolism. Women get more benefits from HIIT than men do.[5] Vary the activity and include weight training for the best long-term results. You'll also see stronger bones and experience reduced bone loss.[6]

You won't have to be a gym rat to see results and other benefits. Only two days per week of upper bodyweight training will show improved memory and cognitive functioning.[7]

Metabolism and Weight Gain

I used to despise walking—why walk when I can run? Kill it and go home. Then, I discovered the many benefits of walking. Walking is like oil for your joints and heart. It burns calories and boosts energy, mood, and muscle tone, not to mention it helps with blood sugar and immunity. Start with a goal that is age- and fitness-level appropriate for you. Try to work up to ten thousand steps daily of purposeful, brisk walking if your doctor agrees.[8]

If you already do a little walking or running, try adding weights. Either hand weights or ankle weights will work. You could even try one of those backpacks you put weights in or a fanny pack. Try doing it twice a week. Even those little one- to five-pound hand weights can make a difference. I have a gym bag of smaller weights, including the ankle strap ones. It's past time I dusted them off and added them to my exercise routine. I added eight-pound weights and could only do one trip around the block.

Talk about multitasking.

Make sure you get enough lean-muscle-making proteins like the ones shown in the list below.

- Almonds and pistachios
- Chicken breast
- Oats
- Greek yogurt
- Broccoli
- Lean beef
- Tuna
- Soybeans and lentils[9]

Be mindful of what goes into your mouth. I'll say it again (as a reminder to myself too): **You cannot out-exercise a bad diet**; you'll end up fit on the outside and dying on the inside, like my plumber.

So, get started.

Do something now.

Talk to your doctor about what diet and exercise regimen might work best for you and any specific needs. If your physician gives you the green light for exercise and you decide to join a gym, many will give you a free consultation with an in-house exercise coach or fitness trainer who will listen to you and create a routine catered to your needs. They will also show you how to use any applicable equipment.

The internet is full of free tutorials and exercise videos you can follow at home too. Recently, I found a few free weight-loss and exercise apps for my phone. The exercise program asked which trouble spots I had. They didn't offer "Select All."

We have to do something to have a better quality of life going into our later years. I for one don't want to shuffle, scooch, and sit, if I can walk, wiggle, and work without aches and pains.

Cholesterol

Women's good cholesterol levels—high-density lipoprotein (HDL)—tend to be higher than men's due to estrogen. The optimum level of about 50 mg/dl enables the good cholesterol to fight the bad, artery-plaque-causing bad cholesterol (LDL). Doctors want the LDL number under 70. They'll add those two numbers to the LDL precursor called very low-density lipoprotein (VLDL) to get your overall number.[10]

Over 200 gets you a caution flag with exercise and dietary recommendations. Over 240 will get you a stern talking to and maybe medications to help bring it down. A doctor will want your triglycerides number under 150 so that this blood fat, in addition to your cholesterol, won't cause artery clogging, which can lead to life-threatening heart conditions or strokes.[11]

Metabolism and Weight Gain

My overall cholesterol has always been high. Sure, I ate a lot of fast food and snacked on chips and dip, but I'd always exercised, too, and had my gymnastics-formed six-pack abs until my forties. As I explained previously, my plumber, the gym rat, ate fast food every day for lunch and succumbed to a fatal heart attack in his mid-fifties. Now I'm the same age and often think about him in association with diet and exercise. Since marrying Dean, my diet has greatly improved, but my total cholesterol is still elevated, usually over 200. However, this year, the tests resulted in a whopping 250 total!

I'd have panicked, but a few years ago, I came across the formula that made my over-200 number OK: total cholesterol divided by HDL. As long as the result is under 5.0, you might get the side-eye from the doctor, but they probably won't put you on medication. Mine came out at 4.55, so I took that as a win but also as a caution since, ideally, the number should be under 3.5.[12]

The struggle gets real as we go through The Change. As our estrogen drops, so does our good cholesterol. With all things, lifestyle and genetics can play a part, but so can diet and exercise. Use the following tips for promoting healthy cholesterol levels.

- Maintain a healthy body weight.
- Don't smoke.
- Exercise for at least 30 minutes five or more days per week.
- Eat a diet rich in fruits, vegetables, lean protein, and high amounts of soluble fiber such as beans and oats, which can reduce LDL.
- Avoid sugar-sweetened drinks and fruit juices—opt for water and unsweetened tea instead—and minimize your intake of other simple carbohydrates like baked goods and candy.
- Drink alcohol in moderation, especially if you have elevated triglycerides.

- Consider the Mediterranean diet, which is rich in fruits, vegetables, grainy breads, and fish. Use olive oil (instead of butter) and spices (instead of salt).
- Eat monounsaturated and polyunsaturated fats—such as those found in olive oil, nuts, and fatty fish like salmon. They can actually have a positive effect on cholesterol, Michos says, by reducing the amount of LDL in the blood and reducing inflammation in the arteries, especially when they replace saturated fats in the diet.

Add these to your shopping list

- Fatty fish such as salmon, trout, mackerel, sardines, and albacore tuna
- Nuts, including walnuts, pecans, almonds, and hazelnuts
- Olive oil to drizzle lightly over your salads and vegetables[13]

A note on the Mediterranean diet: It isn't the same when you use American food. So, grow your own veggies or buy organic with anything with edible skin. (For example, you can buy nonorganic bananas or oranges because you don't eat the peel; apples eaten unpeeled should be organic, as well as berries and grapes. But more importantly, American wheat is much higher in glucose.

Tip: Try ancient wheat grains like einkorn with lower gluten content for bread and pasta instead of modern American (hard husk) wheat. Einkorn wheat and modern European (soft husk) are easier to digest unless you have celiac disease.[14]

CHAPTER 16

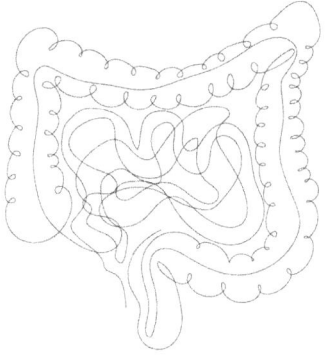

DIGESTIVE ISSUES

Excessive Gas

Passing too much gas? How much is too much? I heard somewhere the average person passes gas a hundred times a day. That sounds like a lot of tooting. For a healthy person, it's more like eight to twenty-five times.[1]

Certain health conditions can increase gas, including IBS, food intolerances, acid reflux conditions, and bacterial overgrowth or intestinal blockage. Sometimes, childbirth can increase gas for months.[2]

As if that's not enough sources, some medications and vitamins can also cause gas. A doctor friend said fish oil supplements could be a culprit. I recently experienced an extreme case and found the cause in an antiaging product I tried. It took me two weeks to figure it out. I always get the bad side effects, never anything good, like looking ten years younger! After two days off those supplements, it subsided. No more orchestra horn sounds announcing my entry and retreat from a room.

Hot Mess Express

If you, too, are careening down the other side of the hill and find yourself reading this book, chances are you can identify with at least one of these conditions. I saw my longtime antagonist, IBS, on the list. What if you didn't see your culprit, but you nonetheless suffer from this embarrassing situation?

Flatulence can usually be alleviated if you quit smoking and chewing gum, limit carbs like pasta and corn, avoid straws and carbonated drinks, and don't lie down after eating. Introduce more insoluble fiber with bran and edible veggie peels, chew foods more carefully, and take more time to eat. Drink more water (hot in the morning with lemon or tea—peppermint or ginger), and exercise daily.[3] Lastly, you can try a heating pad to release any trapped gas.[4]

 Tip: If you're constantly afraid of embarrassing yourself, talk to your doctor. Make a list of your foods and drinks so that you're ready for the visit.

My gas buildup gets so bad at times it doubles me over in pain. I'd welcome a public embarrassment just to get it out. Of course, I'd have to change churches or jobs afterward, but whatever it takes.

My mother enjoys sharing the story of shopping with three-year-old me at the army post exchange, a kind of department store. I writhed in pain and then passed gas. Loudly. "Ah, that's better," she heard me say from under the clothing rack.

Many times, IBS pain comes with an urgent bathroom visit. I've sprinted for the restroom in many places, from department stores to restaurants, even the loathsome gas station. But when the two-minute warning goes off, it doesn't matter if you're unlocking your car door in the mall parking lot or sitting in the living room of the first man you've kissed in twenty years.

Digestive Issues

Time is of the essence if you don't want to have to leave another pair of underwear behind or worry about having a car accident on the way home with your brother's friend responding in the ambulance and finding your unconscious body not wearing bloomers. It did not happen, but the fear of it tormented me.

As did the pain.

I still shopped with my mother decades later, and one of those events happened at a Walmart. Usually, we shopped at a different location, where the female bathroom is to the right as you come around the corner in Customer Service, in the back near televisions. Not so at this particular location.

In my pain and panic, I didn't even look at the door I flung open. Someone else occupied the second stall, so I took the first. During any episode, the pain and expulsion come in waves. So, I waited there for many, many minutes to make sure I finished. During one lull, I scrutinized my neighbor's footwear. Large tan construction boots. Really? I judged them not nearly as fashionable as my tiny size-six-and-a-half Doc Martens.

Then it hit me.

Another wave of panic, but this time not from IBS. I'd finished my business just before I determined a man occupied the next stall. I stopped to wash my hands in the trough sink on the way out. (The only thing worse than being in the wrong bathroom is getting caught not washing after using it.) I hesitated and wondered if I'd just used a urinal to wash in. With the repulsion stifled, I cracked the door and saw no one looking my way. I moved with purpose and found my mother around the corner in the television department.

"That took forever!" she exclaimed.

"We have to leave. I used the wrong bathroom and don't want to be arrested. Let's go!"

All of it comes with IBS. After discussing it with my doctor, she gave me a prescription for Dicyclomine HCL. When it's taken at the first indication of an attack, the soft muscles (colon, intestines) relax. Within twenty minutes, the spasms stop. The bathroom unpleasantness will still happen, but the pain won't be there. I've tried the OTC remedies, like Gas-X, Beano, and Pepto Bismol, but they all failed the IBS challenge.

Trying to reduce carbs from my diet, I bought Colon Pure (psyllium husk, an insoluble fiber) from GNC to make wheat-free bread. The bread wasn't great, so I started drinking it in water with a splash of pomegranate juice. It's the main ingredient in Metamucil, without the sugar or flavor. It worked very well. So well, in our house, we have nicknames for it: "Colon Blow" and "Poo Glue." Like my "Just for Old Ladies" hair regrowth product, it appeared on our Alexa shopping list as one of those nicknames.

However, nothing seemed to come without a price, and my gas increased from taking the psyllium husk. Though insoluble fiber like psyllium is better for constipation and is less likely to cause gas—unlike soluble fiber because it ferments—both can cause bloating and gas.[5] Eventually, I switched to another insoluble fiber product, Citrucel, and experienced less gas. (Soluble fiber is digestible; insoluble fiber is not digestible.)

However, I found the added gas not worth the payoff, so I switched out the powders for a fiber gummy, which produced significantly less noticeable gas than taking no fiber supplements.

 Tip: Check with your doctor before adding fiber supplements to your diet, as it can interfere with medications. Taking prescriptions one hour before or two hours after eating can reduce interference.[6]

Gas can be part of the aging process. Perhaps you're not the little old lady tooting with every step yet, but maybe you don't have to

Digestive Issues

be any day soon or ever. As your metabolism slows, so does the speed at which your food digests, increasing your toot-ilage. Exercise can help you pass gas more quickly and inconspicuously. Certain vegetables, like asparagus, broccoli, and cauliflower (the ABCs of veggies!), can increase gas, but these are a healthy part of your diet, so don't shun them—plan your meals and don't have brussels sprouts or cabbage before a social event.[7]

Beans don't have to be the "musical fruit." To avoid a gas crisis when eating legumes, you can soak the beans overnight. Rinse and change out the water before cooking the next day. Add a teaspoon of baking soda per four quarts or use a safe, modern pressure cooker.[8]

 Tip: Add spices known to help digestion, such as cardamom, cumin, or fennel.[9]

Additionally, to reduce gas, you can decrease dairy or add a digestive aid for dairy sensitivities, avoid constipation, check your medication for digestive side effects, and limit carbonated beverages and high fructose corn syrup.[10]

I'm working on increasing my natural dietary fiber intake. See the list below for suggestions of high-fiber and soluble foods.

Suggested High-Fiber Foods[11]

- Split peas, boiled (1 cup = 16g of fiber)
- Lentils, boiled (1 cup = 15.5g)
- Black beans, boiled (1 cup = 15g)
- Cannellini, Navy, Great Northern beans, canned (1 cup = 13g)
- Chia seeds (1 ounce = 10g)
- Green peas, boiled (1 cup = 9g)
- Raspberries (1 cup = 8g)
- Spaghetti, whole-wheat, cooked (1 cup = 6g)

- Barley, pearled, cooked (1 cup = 6g)
- Pear (1 medium = 5.5g)
- Bran flakes (3/4 cup = 5.5g)
- Turnip greens, boiled (1 cup = 5g)
- Quinoa, cooked (1 cup = 5g)
- Oat bran muffin (1 medium = 5g)

Foods High in Soluble Fiber[12]

- Figs—1.9g per ¼ cup (dried)
- Avocados—13.5g each
- Sweet potatoes—4g each
- Carrots—4.6g per cup (chopped)
- Kidney beans—3g per ¾ cup (cooked)
- Nectarines—2.4g each (medium)
- Apricots—2.1g in 3 apricots
- Guavas—3g each
- Flax seed—3.5g per tablespoon
- Hazelnuts—3.3g per ¼ cup
- Oats—10g per 1¼ cups (dry)

Professionals also suggested starting slowly when adding these fiber-boost wonders to your diet. You could experience extra gas.

Build up so you don't blow up!

Leaky Gut and Lectins

If you have tummy troubles, look into leaky gut and lectins. This is a new area of science. "Leaky gut" is currently still a theory and has yet to be recognized as a medical diagnosis. One theory suggests lectins may be the culprit. Everything has lectins, but some food's lectins may make the intestines more permeable and allow toxins to "leak" into your blood stream. Avoid bad lectins from

Digestive Issues

legumes, nightshades (tomatoes, potatoes, eggplant, and peppers), and whole wheat grains by not eating them raw. Cook them in water or sauce, or bake them.[13]

You can also cut them from your diet, but they have great nutrients. You can choose natural lectin blockers, like cranberries, crustacean shells, kiwi, and pigs' feet, but I didn't care to eat shrimp shells or pigs' feet so haven't incorporated them into my diet and don't plan to any time soon. Instead, I chose a lectin blocker supplement. I took two pills each with my two largest meals of the day to aid in the digestion process.[14]

Regretfully, after four months of using them, I didn't notice any digestive improvement, so I stopped taking them. I have one friend who swears by the supplements, so I encourage you to see if they make a difference for you too.

Poop

To help limit a buildup from gas-producing bacteria, avoid constipation. "Having a bowel movement anywhere from three times daily to once every other day is normal. . . . Hydration and exercise can help keep things moving in this department, too."[15]

Dean once said, "They should put Sally's phone number on the side of the erectile dysfunction medication bottles. If they have an erection lasting four hours or more, they can call her, and she'll talk about her poop until the problem is solved. Works for me every time."

He's not much for bathroom talk, especially from me, which is one of the reasons it took me over half a year to admit I'm doing more in the bathroom than just "pondering life," as I told him after the honeymoon—add a toilet to the statue of *The Thinker* by famous sculptor Rodin, and you've got me. I don't mind talking about it.

Sometimes, you have to stop me from getting too detailed, but I'll try to walk the line for you.

Poop, like most things, can be helped by two things: diet, which includes lots of water, and exercise. The color should be brown, not green, yellow, black, white, or red. Those other colors could mean something is wrong.

The shape is trickier. The best poop is like a hotdog, smooth and soft. If it looks the same, only like your monkey bread fell apart with clear-cut edges, you're still good. This is more likely if you go more than once a day.

If you have separate hard lumps, get more fiber. If your Tootsie Roll poop looks more like a Baby Ruth candy bar, drink more water. A large stool is better than bits; soft is better than hard. And floaters are good since healthy poop takes longer to sink.[16]

CHAPTER 17

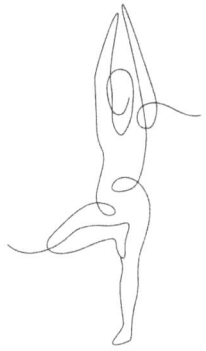

JOINTS

Arthritis and Bursitis

Due to pain, my mother long ago stopped shaking hands. I, too, have experienced pain and swelling in my knuckles during the past two years. From cheerleading, gymnastics, running, and beating my body to a pulp through activities, I also have soreness and stiffness in my hips. No doubt, the extreme activities required in the army also exacerbated the issue.

My gymnastics endeavors took place during my freshmen year of high school. My mother threw me into a regular/weekly beginner's gymnastics class to help me burn off extra energy. She quickly learned the weekly class only gave me more energy, so when the instructor suggested promotion after I'd quickly mastered the class, Mom took her advice and signed me up for the Class IV competition team. We trained four days a week, with a ballet class thrown in on top of Wednesday meetings to instill grace.

Before you get the idea I had superior abilities, please know I did not. I simply found pleasure in something I did well—I caught on quickly. My journey started late at thirteen. I joined the team as the oldest member at fourteen—I led the team only in age but quickly caught up with skills. During that single year, I went from learning how to do a summersault to round-offs, back handsprings, and tucks. We started each practice by assembling the Velcro mats for floor routines and warmups, which consisted of three sets of thirty sit-ups, inverted push-ups against the wall, leg lifts from the high bar, and others I've chosen to forget. At the end of the night, we'd break down the mats and restack them to the side of the community center.

Those mats—maybe you've seen ones like them in your high school gym: blue and a couple of inches thick—seemed to do the trick until we traveled at the end of the season to a private gym for the State of Virginia's Junior Olympics in 1982. (Again, don't be too impressed. Class IV floor exercise routine peaked with a layout dive summersault. Class I had the real gymnasts, like Olympian Mary Lou Retton.) As we warmed up for the event, we discovered the private gym team had a spring floor—actual coil springs, foreign to us, except in our apparatus-mounting springboards used on the beam, bars, and vault. It made the layout dive summersault a lot easier to gain altitude for the layout but harder to roll out of the dive portion as the power we used on our mats caused us to over-rotate on the unfamiliar bouncy floor. Mine were especially brutal to get a handle on with my swayback and me not quite tucking back in from the layout on time. After I'd lost control in midair, I bounced on my butt instead of rolling out smoothly to my feet.

I managed to adapt in time during warm-ups and pulled it off, not with ease, but with enough grace to score decently—enough for seventh place all-around after I'd won a gold medal on the uneven bars and scored well enough on both the vault and balance beam. As I prepared to move up to Class III during the summer of '82, my father got orders to move to Louisiana. We moved to DeRidder, where they had only beginners' gymnastics for the younger ones. The instructor (and high school vice principal's wife) was kind enough to let me use their equipment in our high school's auditorium under my mother's supervision, but to what end? After a few weeks, I quit and enjoyed softball, indoor/outdoor track, and cheerleading. We moved again for my senior year, this time to Hawaii. We'd moved there in time to huddle around the television for the 1984 Olympics. I cheered and watched as Mary Lou Retton finally brought the US women's gymnastics team up to the USSR completion level. She would've crushed them if not for the Soviet boycott; she managed to become our first women's all-around gold medalist. It took the US twenty years to do it again. After a few months in Hawaii, I found a job as an assistant teacher for a beginners' tumbling class—the Keiki Class—for four- and five-year-olds, who did more farting than tumbling. I made it my last year doing anything with gymnastics.

Years later, I saw a commercial with Mary Lou Retton for hip replacement. Since she and I are the same age, a thought came to mind: *Good golly, how old am I?* Only in our mid-thirties I knew it had to be from gymnastics. I felt the effects already in my thirties from gymnastics, cheerleading, and the army, and I'm certain I didn't do half of the body damage she did. As I started thinking my future would include the same, I found out she'd had hip dysplasia, which was compounded by the brutality of gymnastics training at the higher competition level. At least she had the spring floor to help with impact. Without a doubt, it made a huge difference.

Look up a video of a floor routine from the 1968 Olympics and compare it to current floor exercise routines. People didn't simply get better at gymnastics. Yes, skills increased, but those spring floors can make you fly. And if you're fearless, you can do mighty things. In comparison, fear and doubt strangled me, so I'm certain I'd have topped out well before Class II if the army hadn't relocated us.

You don't have to have put your body through the ringer to feel the effects of arthritis. Bursitis is associated with joint inflammation and degeneration of connective tissue and bone and is more common in the hips and knees. It is inflammation of one of the body's more than one hundred fifty bursae. A bursa is a fluid-filled sac-like cavity surrounding joints such as the shoulders, elbows, and big toes.[1]

Arthritis is generally caused by gout or normal wear and tear of the cartilage and connective tissue, leading to bone degeneration, and is associated with the aging process, whereas bursitis is more from trauma, joint infection, or muscle stress. Bursitis can also be caused by autoimmune disorders such as rheumatoid arthritis. You can see arthritis in an X-ray but not bursitis.[2]

Treatment is similar for both arthritis and bursitis: nonsteroidal anti-inflammatory drugs (NSAIDs), such as ibuprofen or naproxen sodium. Doctors also recommend ice and rest and may suggest steroid injections. In severe cases, the bursa may need to be drained or removed.[3]

However, since estrogen helps keep joints, bones, and tendons healthy, I think bioidentical hormone replacement therapy (BHRT), along with a proper diet and weight-bearing exercises, might also benefit this problem. Ask your doctor if this might help you.

Rheumatoid Arthritis and Osteoarthritis

Rheumatoid arthritis (RA), a chronic autoimmune disease, attacks your own healthy tissue, leaving you with pain and joints that no longer work.[4]

Of the 1.5 million people suffering from RA, 70 percent are women. It's what you see in the hands when the joints look swollen and crooked, but it can also wreak havoc on ankles, feet, knees, and other joints. Usually, RA rears its ugly head between the ages of

Joints

forty and sixty and is sometimes called hormonal arthritis. If a parent has it, you may be more susceptible. Symptoms include swelling, stiffness, pain, and redness in any joint, even the jaw.[5]

Often confused with RA, osteoarthritis (OA) impacts approximately twenty-seven million Americans over the age of twenty-five, but mostly the middle-aged to elderly. It's the number-one basis for disability in older age groups.[6]

Though it can stem from genetics, most OA cases result from overuse, abuse, and trauma of the joints. While RA affects the body symmetrically, hitting both sides of the body at the same time, like both knees or wrists, OA does not. It's more random and happens more slowly over time. It increases with physical trauma.[7]

Usually, both RA and OA are treated with over-the-counter anti-inflammatory drugs. Cortisone shots and other drugs can be prescribed for joint pain, which can ease pain and help you move. The more you move, the more you can move. Ironically, though, steroids may be harmful to your joints. Doctors often limit the number of injections you can receive.[8]

 Tip: Exercise can help with arthritis pain and stiffness. It's like greasing the joints.

The changes in barometric pressure land on my face in the form of sinus pressure headaches, but the same inclement weather system can also affect arthritis.

Some people are more sensitive to the weather. Cold, wet climates are known to make arthritis pain worse. This explains the great snowbird migration to my home state of Florida each fall. Barometric pressure changes can aggravate the condition—the cold or warm front coming through your area affects your joints more than the sustained hot or cold weather.[9]

But what about cracking your knuckles? Contrary to old wives' tales, the practice of cracking knuckles is not known to cause arthritis or be harmful in any way.[10]

Cracking your knuckles is merely socially annoying, like snapping or chomping chewing gum.

My arthritic discomfort isn't to the level of shoveling ibuprofen yet, but I'm hedging my bets in the hope that during the next twenty years, science will again make a giant leap and nail down a better cause and discover a cure.

It's pretty bad when your body can outperform the weather forecasters. But I'm cheering on the researchers from the sidelines: "Be . . . aggressive! Be . . . be . . . aggressive, hey!"

Ouch! Hurts to clap, but not from arthritis.

Dupuytren's Contracture

The bumps in the palm of my left hand made handwork uncomfortable. The pea-sized, hard nodule under the skin made clapping in church during praise and worship painful, and they made my white-knuckling steering wheel grip during my work commute almost unbearable. My physician's assistant at the VA's orthopedic clinic thought it might be Dupuytren's Contracture, which is when your fingers start curling into your palm from tissue thickening and forming a cord. The MRI didn't show anything conclusive, but I could feel the bumps.

Naturally, this started in August, and it took until November to see the physician's assistant (PA) in the Veterans Administration's orthopedics department. It took until the end of December to get the MRI, then back to the PA in February. He consulted with the VA orthopedic specialist and referred me for physical therapy in March.

COVID-19 happened, so my late March appointment didn't. They offered to do a tele-visit. I suggested unless they could feel my lumps through the airwaves, we'd better wait until an in-person appointment. They agreed, and finally, in June, they reopened with limited appointments. Thankfully, mine qualified.

Ten months after the bumps came up, the pain subsided. When the therapist checked it out, she had no clue what it might be. I told her only the death grip on the steering wheel during my commute bothered it still, but not as much as initially. Because I had a full range of motion and clapping didn't bother me as much anymore, she set an appointment for a month out.

"You aren't concerned about the bumps?"

"Not really, since it doesn't hurt you so much anymore. We'll have to wait and see if it's Dupuytren's Contracture. Don't forget to call to cancel the appointment if you don't need to come back in."

Treatments for Dupuytren's Contracture include needling—the insertion of a needle to break the cord's contraction. It can be repeated as the condition returns. Enzyme injections can weaken the cord, or there's surgery to remove the tissue. At home, you can cushion your grip surfaces by wearing gloves or using tape on tools or equipment handles. With my eye on a little cheetah print number, I considered a steering wheel grip cover if the bumps got more painful.[11] Thankfully, within months (a year tops), the pain faded away.

Golfer's and Tennis Elbow

Since-yuhs!

"Since I have you here, can you tell me if this is golfer's or tennis elbow?" I showed the physical therapist my right arm.

She had me move in a certain way, then straighten my arm and press against her hand, stopping my movement.

It screamed. "That's the spot."

"Tennis elbow, since it's your outside elbow; golfer's elbow is on the inside."

She showed me how to stretch for both: raise the arm straight in front with the palm facing out like a traffic cop telling you to stop. With your other hand, cup the fingers and pull the hand back toward your face to stretch the bottom of the forearm, which is the wrist extensor stretch. Then, let the hand drop with the arm still straight and pull against the back of the hand toward your body to stretch the top of the forearm (wrist flexor stretch). Hold each of these for fifteen seconds and repeat three times.

"Let me get approval, and I'll send you home with a tennis elbow brace." She returned again with the brace. "At least your trip wasn't a waste."

"Thank you, though I'd hoped for more of an answer. The PA already said it wasn't cancer, but I just wanted to see if you had any other ideas."

"I'm sorry, I don't. Wish I did." She walked me out.

I did cancel the appointment the next month because the painful bump lessened to the point where I forgot it existed. With the stretching exercise, the discomfort of the tennis elbow subsided too.

Occasionally, the arm pain returns, and I do my stretches. Also, as my chiropractor showed me, I have Dean rub the tendon from wrist to elbow in one smooth action.

 Tip: Without intervention, both golfer's and tennis elbow will go away on their own within a year, but stretching will cut the time severely.

Shoulders

My left shoulder screamed when I reached too high or grabbed something with my arm extended to the side. It started one spring and worsened to the point where I had to have Dean help with taking fitted dresses and shirts off. I remember one dress in particular, a cute traditional Chinese dress I'd picked up in China while staying with a missionary family in 2003. Yes, it'd been a few days since I'd tried it on, but I wanted to wear it to a family wedding in Vegas. I wanted to make sure it still fit; it did not. The fitted dress with zero give or stretch only went on over my head but wouldn't go over the chest and shoulder region, and I couldn't put it in reverse, with my left shoulder useless. In my precarious situation, I called for Dean, who fared well, stifling his laughter enough to extricate me.

Another dress arrived like magic on the front porch, and I flew to my niece's wedding. One afternoon, I hung with my sister and some of the thirty-something "kids" as we ran around The Strip getting social media–worthy photos. In one casino, we ambled around, trying to find the Excalibur Knight. We finally found it hidden in an obscure alcove, got our pics, and happily made our way back toward our hotel.

In an open area near the lobby, two of the younger guys tried to do a cartwheel. My sister eyed me and held her hand out to hold my water. Much in the fashion of "hold my beer," I handed her my water and purse. She yelled at them to behold a proper cartwheel, and I obliged. But on the way back to the standing position, my shoulder screamed. From the overwhelming pain, I'd lost the ability to stand. I held onto consciousness and waited it out from the casino floor. Eww, I know.

The wedding trip happened over Labor Day. By October, I could no longer sleep on that side. I had pain from any surprise jerk or twitch, like when Dean played one of our favorite games of stealthfully entering a room and suddenly appearing right in front of me. During that point, a surprise scream and a painful cry follow the violent twitch from surprise. Afterward, he tried to minimize those events by announcing his arrival in any part of the house, like a leper in biblical times, "Unclean! . . . Unclean!" But I'm so jumpy,

I'd twitch or jerk even when he didn't intend to surprise me. We'll call it a lack of sleep.

I would forget it was an issue until I moved it the wrong way, and the pain came in waves. At first, I couldn't breathe, and I couldn't move. For twenty to thirty seconds, my world came to a complete stop. My vision narrowed. Then it passed, and I could breathe again.

I cried uncle to the VA in late October, and they sent me to X-ray, then on to physical therapy, which didn't help. By mid-January, I qualified for an MRI, which they called for in February and scheduled an April appointment. Dr. W., my chiropractor, conjectured an impinged shoulder and sent me to check out Bob and Brad's physical therapy YouTube videos to help me discern between impinged shoulder and rotator cuff injury. He said I'd know them when I found them. (He wasn't wrong.) I couldn't narrow it down and didn't want to wait another four months until the VA's MRI appointment, so I booked an appointment with an outside provider and paid cash—just under $300.

While I sat against a wall in the inner waiting area, I watched the techs each work the two MRI machines and waited for my turn. My technician turned to me and asked what I did to my shoulder.

"I'm not sure exactly because it didn't come on suddenly. It's gotten worse over the months since last spring." And then it hit me. "I think it might've been the HIIT workout with weights . . . out to the side . . . side lateral raise." I demonstrated, kind of.

He shook his head. "You're not meant to do that."

"But I only had three- or five-pound weights in each hand. And the guy is a professional trainer."

"Nope. Do you know how many people I see for MRIs because of that?" He then explained forward and backward motions only, especially with weights, but not to the side.

Ugh. Undone trying to do the right thing. Again.

Joints

When I forwarded the MRI results to the VA, they got me in with a specialist two months later. She said the pain stemmed from an impinged shoulder, just as Dr. W. had suggested months before. She recommended a cortisone shot to calm the inflamed bursa sac. I got the shot the next week and then again two months later in July, along with one in my right shoulder, which had been taking the brunt of everything for the past fifteen months.

It's been another six months, and the right shoulder has settled down mostly. But the left shoulder is still bothersome, though I can dress myself now, and the screaming has stopped in my shoulder and from me. I still stretch it and hang from the bar occasionally, as instructed. But as I sat down to write this portion, I stopped and wondered if I could do a push-up again. Yes, I cranked out two. It's been a day, as the kids say.

Next test, cartwheel.

Word on the internet street is frozen shoulder isn't caused by menopause directly, but it's suspected low estrogen affecting bones, cartilage, and inflammation are indirectly to blame, with two-thirds of those suffering being female and between forty and sixty.[12] With reduced bone density, muscle and tendons weaken, leaving women more vulnerable to joint pain and damage during the menopause years.[13]

Frozen shoulder results from fibroid tissues forming on the joint, causing pain and stiffness. There are three stages: the freezing stage, when pain is severe, and motion is reduced; the frozen stage, which includes reduced pain and continued decreased range of motion; and then the thawing stage, when it finally returns to normal. All of this typically takes one to three years for the complete cycle.[14]

Sometimes, the shoulder freezes after immobilization due to an injury, like a broken or sprained arm in a sling for weeks. For those cases, physical therapy can help with stretching and strengthening exercises. When there is no trauma cause, diet and exercise can help, but doctors often recommend HRT with estrogen as the focus.[15]

It makes total sense that with declining estrogen levels, joints and bones could be affected. This then begs the question of why women are not tested and treated for lowering hormones before something bad happens. Why aren't we tested for baseline when all is well and then periodically as we age? I will tell you part of the answer is, as I've heard a few women doctors lately explain on social media, that medical students spend only a few hours on the topic of aging women during their four years of medical school. One brave doctor explained that they learned nothing after a woman's child-bearing years and have to self-teach. Almost all testing and teaching about aging is for men's health.

CHAPTER 18

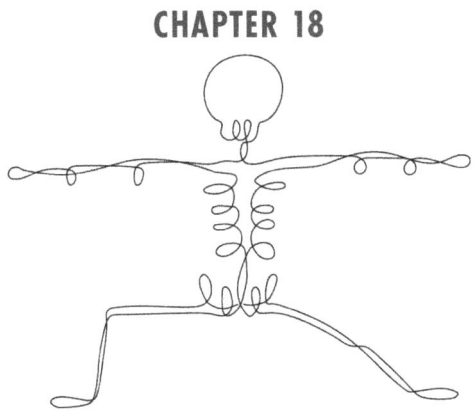

BONES

Osteoporosis

When I was fifty-four years old, while roller-skating with the nieces, Dean warned me not to fall or I could break a hip at my age—just his reminder I'm a whole four months older than he is. I fell three times, each time with my feet straight out and onto my rump with hands out to the side. Weeks later, I'd noticed my wrists weren't healing right. Two months later, while waiting on a COVID-19-era teleappointment with my VA general practitioner to discuss the wrists, I'd grabbed wrapping paper from the attic. While shutting the access door, my middle finger caught in the rope's loop as it slammed shut. My doctor ordered X-rays of my wrists and finger, along with a bone density scan (DEXA).

We did the X-ray, and the technician asked me to follow him to the next test. I didn't realize the doctor had ordered the DEXA scan. I hopped up on the table, and the technician stood there with confusion written all over his face. "Let me guess, you usually have to help the patients onto the table?"

Of course, he did. The tech commented how I'm by far the youngest he'd done a DEXA scan on.

The wrists weren't broken, but the results did show a fracture in the finger. The scan results showed osteopenia, a lessening of minerals in the bones (bone mineral density—BMD), a precursor to osteoporosis.

I should stop saying how I identify as a ninety-two-year-old man before my self-fulfilling prophecies also give me a man's prostate problem.

Osteoporosis is a greater concern for women than men as we age. This condition is marked by the body's inability to keep up with the constant natural breaking down and remaking of bone tissues. The resulting fractures, typically in the hips, spine, and wrists, can be caused by as little as a cough or other ordinary movements.[1]

How many times have we heard of an older woman taking a spill and breaking a hip? Half of all women over the age of fifty will break a bone due to low bone density. (My chiropractor says at ninety, you don't fall and break a hip; your hip breaks, and then you fall.) In less than twenty minutes, your doctor can do a DEXA scan to measure your bone density.

The weakening of the bone is more prevalent in women over fifty. Even healthy people lose bone density after the age of thirty-five. Healthy bones naturally break down and then rebuild. As we age, the bones rebuild more slowly. This causes a loss of overall bone over time. Your doctor will assess your loss rate to determine if you have a problem.

Causes of Osteopenia[2]

- Medical conditions such as hyperthyroidism.
- Medications such as prednisone and some treatments for cancer, heartburn, and seizures.

Bones

- Hormonal changes during menopause.
- Poor nutrition, especially a diet too low in calcium or vitamin D.
- Unhealthy lifestyle choices, such as smoking, drinking too much alcohol or caffeine, and not exercising.

Your orthopedic specialist can track your BMD and treat it with medication to help slow the bone breaking down. Since low levels of estrogen are usually the culprit, hormone replacement therapy for estrogen with either pills or a patch is an option.[3] Doctors can use hormones or bisphosphonate pills. Injected medications are reserved for extreme cases.[4]

In addition to estrogen, try weight-bearing or resistance exercises, walking, and climbing stairs. You can also see improvements with good nutrition. To slow the downhill roll, eat foods rich in calcium, like dairy, and increase vitamin D in your diet. Quit smoking and limit alcohol to one drink per day to see the best results.[5]

Tip: Women over fifty should have a diet with daily servings of calcium (1,200 mg) and vitamin D3 (600 IU/800 IU after the age of 70) with vitamin K2 (80mg), which helps the body absorb the calcium and then get it from the blood into your bones.[6] Since these recommendations can change often, check with your doctor for current recommended amounts.

The VA doctor suggested I start with calcium supplements. After about a year of taking them, I learned the body doesn't absorb the supplements like it does the calcium in foods. There isn't enough research to suggest the nutrient pills help, but there are studies linking them to cancerous colon polyps, kidney stones, and heart disease because the body can't absorb more than five hundred milligrams daily from pills. The rest floats around, causing trouble. I took more than twice that amount.[7] Stick to a calcium-rich diet and weight-bearing exercises instead. Here are a few examples of calcium-rich foods.

- Seeds—poppy seeds, sesame seeds
- Cheese—parmesan, cheddar
- Yogurt
- Fish—sardines, salmon
- Beans/Lentils
- Almonds
- Whey protein
- Leafy greens—collards, spinach, kale
- Rhubarb
- Amaranth (seeds and leaves)
- Edamame/Tofu
- Figs (dried)
- Milk[8]

Those with osteoporosis should avoid twisting at the spine and bending at the waist, especially in their exercises. Avoid sports such as golf. See your doctor for alternatives.[9]

Good bone health comes right back to diet and exercise. The consensus for testing is at the age of sixty-five for women. Again, I'm left wondering why the medical world still hasn't caught on. Wouldn't earlier testing catch osteopenia before it advances to osteoporosis and allow us more time to make the changes we need for healthier bones? If you feel strongly about this, you can advocate for yourself. Be brave. Switch doctors if you run up against a wall or are treated like you're crazy.

My mother's doctor tests her regularly and prescribes medication for stronger bones. Genetics—it's no wonder I, too, will now get tested regularly and have to address my diet and exercise routines, or one day, like Mom, I may also be prescribed medication. At least

Bones

they caught mine early. Genetics can only suggest tendencies; you have the power to override your own lifestyle deficiencies.

Perhaps I'll start taking after my father's side, but it would be another load of problems, starting with how they all seem to decline early but linger for decades in a decrepit state. So, never mind.

In addition to bones becoming more brittle as we age due to bone density loss, they make us look funny too. Arm and leg bones get more brittle with age, but they don't shrink like the torso, so you have arms that look too long.[10] My midsection started out disproportionately shorter than my limbs. Oh, am I going to be funny-looking.

I can't wait to look like George's dad on *Seinfeld*. "Serenity, now!"

The expectations of looking like an alien are not welcomed. I seriously need to increase my calcium and vitamin D intake. And those hand weights won't lift themselves.

CHAPTER 19

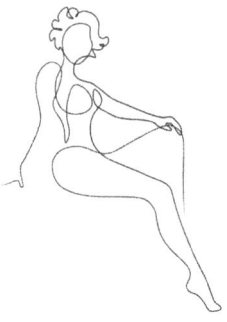

HEALING

My first attempt at college started in the fall of 1985. I pulled the plug on the party at the end of the fall quarter in 1986. During those months of not enough study and too much fun, I hung out at a house nicknamed The Cove. The guys who lived there had built a half-pipe for skateboarding. They called me a Skate Betty—she who oohs and ahs at the skater's eggplants, ollie-over-the-channel, and other tricks.

One of the guys began college after four years in the military. He hobbled around on his crutches when I first met him. After a couple of months, he again skated the half-pipe with the eighteen- and nineteen-year-olds. His injury is the first thing I think about when I ponder the effects of aging on the body's ability to heal. He'd admitted at the ripe old age of twenty-five that he could already see a difference in the amount of time it took his body to heal compared to eighteen, let alone fourteen.

Yes, once you injure yourself, you are more likely to reinjure the same area. At least for pulls, sprains, and strains. As we age, the amount of time it takes to heal increases. Scientists don't know why, but they have their theories.

One doctor suggested three culprits as possible explanations of why we take more time and sometimes incompletely recoup: elevated inflammatory response, cell exhaustion, and the changing biochemical environment.[1]

Each injury brings an inflammatory response in the body. The inflammatory cells may not perform as well as we age; the regulation of those cells is lacking. Sometimes, there's too much inflammation or not enough to heal properly. Other muscle stem-cell-like repair assistants may be compromised in their ability to replicate themselves. Then, as hormonal levels change with age, muscular healing is impaired.[2]

A surgeon intimated that older people may have a hard time reconciling the fact that they no longer have youth on their side and jump into new activities that are too robustly causing injuries.[3]

My roller-skating incident proved his theory. I also pulled my hip flexors while doing exercises I've done in years past, but it'd been a while since the last time, and I didn't go into it incrementally.

The same surgeon also conjectured that the healing process is waylaid by a decrease in growth hormones. Sometimes, children break bones and heal without intervention, whereas an older adult might need surgery for the same injury. Your body's clock is slowing down.[4]

As discussed in chapter 8, "Skin," thinning skin shows bruising more readily, and the healing process slowing down makes it take longer to disappear. Wounds take longer to heal too. In bites, cuts, scrapes, and scratches, a scab forms to protect the wound from infection, while new skin cells form underneath. It's why they say, "Don't pick the scab!" As the wound heals, new tissue forms, closing the wound and repairing the cells underneath the scab. As we age, the process gets slower and sometimes doesn't complete.

Healing

Reduced skin elasticity means older people have a higher chance of wound scarring. Slower collagen replacement hinders wound healing too. In addition, older people have a higher chance of developing conditions like cardiovascular disease, diabetes, and other blood-flow issues, which make healing more difficult.[5]

A healthy diet of protein, fruits, vegetables, dairy, and grains strengthen the healing process. Certain vitamins and minerals can boost healing, like vitamin C and zinc.[6] (See your doctor before starting supplements.)

Dietary improvements can go a long way in recovery. You can also add heat to improve blood flow to the area, elevate the wound area, stop smoking, and get moving. Exercise will help you recover more quickly, but you don't want to push it and reopen a wound.[7]

The more you do, the more you *can* do.

Moving correctly will help you avoid further injuries elsewhere. When I hurt my ankle, my chiropractor told me to stop limping, or it would throw my back out further. When we hurt ourselves below the hips, we tend to favor the injured leg. It throws our gate or stride off, causing problems elsewhere in the body. Be careful and listen to your doctor, but as best as you can, keep your gate normal.

Tip: My chiropractor told me he sees more people at Christmastime after they've wrapped presents while sitting on the floor. Instead, stand at a countertop or table. The less leaning, the better.

CHAPTER 20

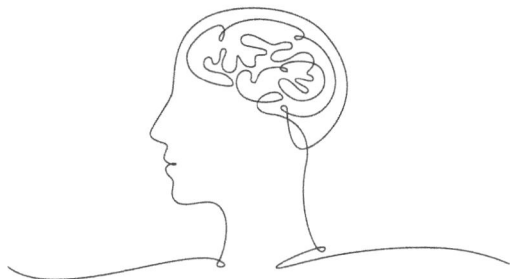

THE BRAIN

A loved one once said to me, "If I ever get to that point, just shoot me."

It's hard to imagine. I don't ever want to deal with a scrambled brain in an immediate family member or myself, but I hope I'd have the grace to do either well. It feels like a foreboding cloud stalking us all.

As we age, the brain shrinks, increasing the chances of stroke, lesions, and dementia. The digressions affect blood flow and cognition. Memories fade with the decreasing levels of neurotransmitters and hormones. Diet and exercise positively impact the brain's functions, along with decreasing alcohol consumption. Continued learning or working in a job or career can help, too—anything that keeps you problem-solving.[1]

We are all painfully aware of how brutal the latter stages of life can be. Most of us have watched a loved one deteriorate from stroke, dementia, or other brutal diseases, which wasted away their brain and body. We've seen it in the movies. We've heard friends talk about their parents or grandparents. If you're anchored in this life and not an orphaned drifter, you've seen this.

I want to give you some hope for the future, but first, the nitty-gritty.

Cognitive Changes

Some of the common struggles in thinking as we age are searching for the right word or remembering names, multitasking, and paying attention.[2]

I've had those problems my entire life. As previously mentioned, the VA tested me for attention deficit disorder (ADD/ADHD). In the end, they came up short and suggested I simply have issues or struggles in those areas, but not to the level at which they could label me with a diagnosis. Don't we all have issues, especially in this microwave society, where everybody wants stuff now and with everything distracting us and vying for our attention?

So, wait . . . where was I? Oh, yeah.

How will my loved ones ever know if I'm slipping away or just displaying my usual absentmindedness?

Degrees, I suppose.

Here's the good news: science makes advancements in the study of the aging brain all the time. Doctors are constantly learning more. Evidence shows the brain remains malleable as we age, leaving us the ability to rise to new tests and trials.[3]

Memory

A memory study reported that researchers tracked thousands of neurons during memory pairing testing. (Are you thinking of the card game Concentration?) The neurons fired in the same pattern right before the person remembered those same pairs.[4]

The Brain

Scientists have even discovered a gene affecting memory as much as night and day. Literally, the time of day can influence memory recall. Have problems recollecting? Write it down and revisit the matter later in the day.[5]

Of course, the opposite is true with dementia patients. "Sundowning" is the term for the late-day confusion compounded by the diminishing daylight. Those suffering seem to be cognizant earlier in the day.[6]

Another study connected the addition of a specific amino acid nutritional supplement with reducing memory loss for Alzheimer's sufferers, repairing early affected spatial memory.[7]

Remember the story of Pavlov's dog, who learned by conditioning or repetition? When Pavlov paired food with the sound of a bell, the dog eventually would salivate at just the sound of the bell—even without food being presented. Conditioning. Well, researchers have found the neurons involved. The neurons act in concert when a new memory forms, like a few synchronized swimmers in a crowded pool.[8]

Four recent groundbreaking studies in only six months give me lots of hope.

A recent discovery also led to a better understanding of how Alzheimer's and a decline in cognitive ability affect an aging brain. Scientists discovered lymphatic vessels surrounding the brain, which scientists previously said did not exist. These are the brain cleaners.

With the use of a compound, they were able to enlarge the vessels, causing them to drain better in mice. They further applied it to Alzheimer's and found if they blocked the vessels, then amyloid plaques associated with Alzheimer's built up. Researchers admit it's still hard to reverse Alzheimer's, but they might be able to delay the initial onset until much later.[9]

Elsewhere, because of the plaque buildup, scientists are thinking they can use a marijuana compound to remove toxic Alzheimer's protein from the brain. The THC (tetrahydrocannabinol) in marijuana helps eliminate toxic clumps of amyloid-beta protein in the brain, which are thought to usher in the disease.[10]

Doctors are now referring to Alzheimer's as diabetes type 3 or diabetes of the brain. Just as diabetes causes damage to the body by impairing blood vessels and restricting the flow of nutrients, it's doing the same in the brain. They further declared type 2 diabetics are at a higher risk of Alzheimer's.[11]

Along with having to give up sweets, they may be losing function in portions of the brain.

The 2017, trials produced positive results when they used an insulin nasal inhaler, which slowed or even improved cognitive deterioration.[12]

We've come a long way in diagnosing and studying the aging brain. I am hopeful that, in my lifetime, we will see cures and preventative measures discovered.

Brain Fog

Brain fog happens—bad nutrition, sleep issues, stress, and workload can affect your brain function. Most of us have experienced going into a room and forgetting why, misplacing keys or important papers, or inability to recall a common word—even when you can see an image in your mind!

Again, I've suffered from this most of my life, but lately, it intensifies on Fridays—aside from COVID-19, where every day seemed like Friday for about six months. I'm exhausted from a lack of quality sleep and can't think properly. As I said in chapter 4, "Insomnia," I will never own another multilevel house unless the master is on the ground level. You can only forget something upstairs so many times before you become disgusted with yourself.

The Brain

See your doctor for help identifying underlying causes, like medication side effects and medical conditions. But if there is no other reason for the inability to remember things normally recalled or the sudden lack of reasoning skills, you can probably blame it on your hormonal changes. I'm chalking yet another burnt dinner up to brain fog. I set numerous timers and still ended up with a disappointing meal. Crockpot meals are easier. You don't have to pay attention; set it and forget it.

As much as it is up to you, get enough good-quality sleep. Cognitive function and alertness are benefits of a proper night's rest. Along with diet and exercise, drinking enough water and likewise decreasing any diuretic such as caffeine is recommended to ease symptoms of brain fog.[13]

Ability to Learn Declines

Our ability to learn slows as we age. I think mine slowed in my twenties and came to a screeching halt in my forties.

The ability to learn a new language with the proficiency of a native speaker diminishes after the age of eighteen, and it's beneficial if you start learning the language by the age of ten.

So, what hope do we have?

You can still learn a language at any point in your life, but not with the aptitude you once could. You can always learn a new trick, and the process of learning new hobbies or skills helps keep your mind in shape.[14]

You peak in different areas throughout your life. At different ages, from eighteen to sixty-seven, we reach the apex of various learning endeavors. In my mid-fifties, I've already peaked in tracking details, catching names and new faces, concentrating, and others. At this point, I'd better get on with acquiring new vocabulary before that caps off at around age sixty-seven.[15] See the list below for more skills and the ages at which they peak.

- 18—we peak at brain processing power and keeping track of details.
- 22—learning unfamiliar names
- 32—learning new faces
- 43—concentrating
- 48—reading others' emotions
- 50—understanding/learning new information and arithmetic/overall knowledge
- 67—vocabulary[16]

I always figured as you aged, you pushed out valuable information when you tried to cram more in. Not quite, but you are declining in certain areas, even as you increase in others. At least, until a certain age, then it all declines.[17] But you can control to what extent, somewhat.[18]

Satisfaction, Self-Love, and Agreeability Peak Later in Life

Certain skills, like a nice wine, can get better with time, even well into middle age or later. A German study found that even though twenty-three-year-olds are particularly happy with their lives, it peaks again at sixty-nine.

A Gallup survey stated body confidence through self-love and acceptance peaked past the age of retirement, along with wisdom. In another study, retirees gave the highest level of psychological well-being, peaking between eighty-two and eighty-five.[19]

More good news is that psychologists now believe personalities are not fixed. People tend to become more disciplined and organized. They also become more congenial as they enter the twilight years.[20]

The Brain

The image of the old man shaking his fist while yelling "Get off my grass" at the kids playing is not the picture of a typical older person. Though I often identify with him, we don't have to become him. We can still make friends, work a paying job, create and innovate, and some things we can do better than the young whippersnappers.

Never Too Late to Learn a New Trick

The more you do, the more you *can* do. It does not apply only to physical fitness but also to mental fitness. Learning new skills keeps the mind sharp—actual skills, not just crossword, Sudoku, or puzzles.[21]

My mother once said, "You sure do go to school a lot for someone who never liked school." She wasn't wrong. And I hate learning new things. I still struggle with the idea of new information pushing out the old, and I like some of the old material. It's never been easy to remember something I wanted to recall, but now I see the importance of challenging the mind, even if it frustrates me.

 Tip: If you take the easy path, you won't grow, you won't renew, and you won't even maintain the knowledge you already have.

In the previously mentioned study of older adults learning new tricks, they offered new skills, including learning a new language. They found that older adults can acquire many new skills simultaneously, which improves their overall cognitive functionality. Additionally, it made them feel more confident about new challenges.[22]

So, get on it!

In the middle of writing this book, I switched my computer mouse to my left hand. It wasn't easy to retrain myself, but I think it checks off the box of increasing my cognitive function. Nobody around me has noticed the new improved me yet, but maybe when I can finally get a decent night's sleep, it will become more apparent.

Time Flies

Does time fly when you're having fun? Of course, but it also flies more as you get older. As I get older, the days seem shorter. Not so in my younger days, when Mom told us to be home when the street lights came on. The hours we played around the neighborhood seemed like an eternity. So did church and school. The hours felt like days; now, the days feel like hours. Beyond the fact those days were indeed simpler times, every day we get closer to death—all of us—but there's a scientific explanation for why time seems to pass more quickly as we get older.

A study compared how many more images a baby's eyes process than an older adult's eyes. The aging nerves and neurons slow the brain's imaging speed, giving the illusion of time speeding up.[23]

As we age, our brain's nerves and neurons slow the flow of electrical signals. Consequently, new mental images and memories are gathered, processed, and stored more slowly, too, which makes time seem like it's going by more quickly.

They pointed to babies' rapid eye movements as evidence of their quick processing.[24]

Just one more reason to coo over the wee little ones.

CHAPTER 21

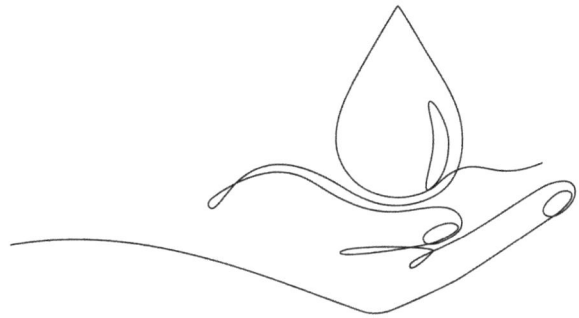

DEHYDRATION

Recently, I went to the lab for more hormone tests. Déjà vu gripped me when I ended up with the same tech who'd previously used me as a pin cushion. As before, she jabbed around and then passed me on to Frank, who got the job done. Again.

Frank rebuked me. "You're dehydrated."

I grunted. "I don't drink enough, I know. But I don't get it; I drank extra water last night and this morning before coming in."

"Did you sip or gulp?" He stared at the vial, waiting for my answer as the blood finally started its slow lavalike flow.

My brain searched for the correct answer—like back in school when I thought there wasn't necessarily a correct answer, only what the teacher wanted me to say. I made my best second guess. "Gulp?"

Wrong.

"You need to sip. You know when you see on the news or in a movie some poor guy rescued from the desert, and the paramedics give him water and tell him to sip not gulp?"

"Yeah, but I thought it was so they didn't throw up."

Hot Mess Express

Frank skillfully switched out yet another vial. "Partially, but mostly, it's because when you gulp, your body expels most of that. More water gets absorbed when you sip."

When the needle clogged with thick clotted blood, he started a new butterfly needle in my hand for the final two of eleven vials. That made six sticks in all, including the attempts by she-who-shall-not-be-named.

Seriously, why hadn't I heard about sip versus gulp during the past half-century?

Exercise and diet are key components of good health and weathering the effects of menopause in its various stages. As part of our bad diets, many of us run around in various stages of dehydration. We all learned in school that the earth is 70 percent covered in water. Our bodies, likewise, are largely water—vital to all plants and animals.

H_2O affects all parts and functions of the human body. Adam Sandler's Waterboy knew of its importance. I harped in previous chapters on the need to drink enough water. But it's of such significance it deserved a whole chapter for emphasis.

Recommendations about water consumption are all over the place. Should you drink eight cups a day? Not necessarily. Should you be drinking more than that? Maybe, maybe not. Can you drink too much water? Absolutely. Water intake is different for men versus women, for active versus inactive, for those who live in the arctic versus those who live along the equator. The National Academy of Medicine (NAM) recommends consuming ninety to one hundred twenty ounces (eleven to fifteen cups) of water per day, including what we get from other drinks and food. But NAM also acknowledges that making broad recommendations is not ideal for everyone for the reasons just listed.[1] Basically, they say drink to quench your thirst. That should meet your basic fluid needs. It's also important to note that other parts of our diet are working against us, like caffeine

Dehydration

and alcohol, which expel fluids from our bodies. It's probably best to minimize or cut these items.

Maybe you're like me and just get busy and forget. Even with a twenty-four-ounce cup at the ready, I'd only consumed half by the end of the workday. Then, at home with a filled travel mug of water, I'd find most of it remaining at bedtime. Not only that, but what I did drink, I mostly gulped with vitamins and fiber gummies at dinnertime.

We know gulp: it's chug, guzzle, and swig. But what is a sip? Try taking a mouthful of water, leaving room to swish it around, then slowly swallow. Think of it like a wine tasting. Savor it. Add flavor if you don't like plain water. (Try an app like Yuka or Bobby Approved to find one that's healthy.) Try a sip once every ten minutes to see how far that gets you on your way to hydration. Adjust as necessary. Additionally, we slowly dehydrate overnight. So, it's important to start after you wake up each morning.

So, how do we get that needed water sipped daily?

Determination. Make up your mind to do it. Determine to make water intake a priority. Give your spouse, friends, or others permission to hold you accountable. Baby steps. Don't be too hard on yourself.

Intentionality. Keep water handy at all times. Have some in your car during your morning commute, on your desk, by your seat in the evenings, or nearby when you exercise. And keep some on the nightstand. Don't gulp it at bedtime, but if you end up getting up to go to the bathroom during the night, take a sip of water.

Persistence. If you fail to drink enough water during the day, give yourself grace and start again. Keep at it until you've built the new habit. Set reminders hourly and daily, and then monthly to see if you're still on track or need to reset mentally.

If it can work for me, it can work for you. I set my mind to getting hydrated, and I saw the difference in my next lab visit three months later. I sat in a chair with an unknown phlebotomist, nervous about being the test subject again. When I bravely glanced over to check the progress of the first vial, the tech had already filled five and was working on the final tube. I'd never seen it flow so quickly. No more lava, tar, or crude oil oozing out. And no more human pincushion—one stick and done.

Frank walked by, and I thanked him. I shared how I'd implemented his advice. He said I was the only woman who ever listened to him.

Fear can also be a useful motivator. Dehydration is present in 60 percent of stroke patients. One study says it may be a contributing factor.[2] Strokes also seem to be skewed toward the elderly with too many on the commode.[3] Dehydration is also thought to be the cause of more severe symptoms and delayed healing.[4] Elvis Presley, the most famous American to die on the toilet, died at forty-two. Granted, he had a massive opioid problem, which caused constipation. We won't know the official cause of his death until 2027, when his autopsy is unsealed. However, constipation can be greatly helped with an adequate amount of daily water along with fiber.

Avoid straining to poo. Use a step stool to raise your legs to relax certain muscles and make it easier to go. Don't force it. Dehydration can back up blood in narrowed blood vessels. Straining can exacerbate the issue and trigger a stroke or heart attack, especially if you've already been diagnosed with clogged arteries.[5] Breathe through any pushing, just like childbirth. Better yet, just go sip some water and come back later when you have the urge to move your bowels.

Exercise can help you poo too. When I got tired of making mental contingency plans every time, like when I saw a big bush to squat behind or an alleyway to duck into, I altered my running route to make sure I could be home ASAP if my IBS kicked in. Running seemed to encourage the bowels to move. Quickly. "Hey,

Dehydration

there's another spot if I can't make it home in time." You can only poop your pants so many times before it chips away at your soul.

If you consistently fail to reach your daily water goals, you can also drink low-fat milk, herbal tea, juices, and broth-based soups.[6] You'll also get fluids that count with the high water content already in the following foods:

- Lettuce: 96% water
- Celery: 95% water
- Zucchini: 95% water
- Cabbage: 92% water
- Watermelon: 91% water
- Cantaloupe: 90% water
- Honeydew melon: 90% water[7]

Drinking coffee and sodas throughout the day reminds me of what a doctor told me decades ago, and it stuck with me. "Drink plenty of water. It cleanses your insides. You wouldn't take a shower in coffee or sodas, would you?"

No, Doc, I would not.

Being fully hydrated can help with digestion and weight loss. It'll keep your bowel movements more regular, cutting down on those associated irritations like gas, bloating, and heartburn. Drinking more water can help you feel fuller and cut down on snacking. It helps your heart pump oxygen, so you'll feel more energetic. Adding extra water aids the brain with cognition, lowering anxiety and regulating emotions. Water is lubrication for the joints and helps your body temperature regulate better.[8]

Furthermore, adequate hydration helps prevent kidney stones and helps regulate your body's detox system. Want fewer headaches? That's right, water is the answer to that one too.

You can live weeks without food, but the human body only survives about three days without water.

CHAPTER 22

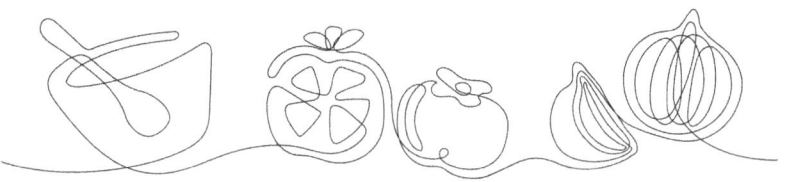

WHAT IS *DIET*?

Try to think of *diet* as a way to live your life rather than a temporary sacrifice to lose weight. Everybody is different, so we react differently to various foods. Talk to your doctor about eating better and any special needs you'll have to consider.

When I listen to various speakers talk about their ideal diet, I try to imagine a Venn diagram with overlapping circles to see what they all have in common. What do they agree is bad for you? And where is there a consensus in what is healthy?

Perhaps a nutritional, intellectual cage match is called for as there is so little agreement among experts. If only we could gather traditional medical doctors, holistic doctors, biologists, and other more modern nutritional gurus and put them all on the same platform to hash it out.

I did a deep dive into nutrition so you wouldn't have to. You're welcome. My head spun for months, and I feel like I've done enough studying to get an advanced degree.

Some experts I read about used a study from the 1970s or 1980s, and others shot them down with a study from within the last decade. One study on a topic is interesting, but two or more studies with the same results raise my attention—now I'm listening. Otherwise, studies and statistics can be twisted to say what the presenter wants them to say, especially if it supports their opinion, so I look for consensus on any topic.

Sometimes, you only need to look at the reaction of an industry.

The Sugar Debate and Marketing

A study on sugar said it stimulates the pleasure and reward pathways in the brain.[1] (Some think it's comparable to cocaine in addictiveness.) I think the food industry believes that study to be true and why it's so hard to find a bottled or boxed product made without sugar.[2]

A 2013 study showed that rats preferred Oreo cookies over cocaine and morphine. The fat and sugar of the delectable cookies lit up the pleasure center of their brains significantly more than did the drugs. They also cracked open the Oreos to eat the middle first, like we do.[3]

Most experts warn of "added sugar," hidden in plain sight in foods like soda, fruit drinks, and ready-to-eat cereals. And a sugar by any other name should be shunned as well: brown sugar, corn syrup, high-fructose corn syrup, honey, and tree syrup.[4] They hide in granola and power bars too.[5] Sugar is addicting, and all added sugars are inflammatory.[6]

You can find a few processed foods with healthier sugar substitutes by looking for monk fruit, stevia, and erythritol as the sweetener. Those sweeteners don't spike on the glycemic index, though erythritol has been linked to some other health concerns.[7] It's best to eliminate all added sugar and get your body's necessary sugar from natural sources like whole foods in moderation, such as fruit, dairy, and grains.[8]

What Is *Diet*?

With this new knowledge in mind, I set out to eliminate sugar from my diet. During the next trip to the grocery store, I went armed with two food nutritional phone apps, Yuka and BobbyApproved (BA). I opened the apps and hit the scan features. Yuka helped me begin to reign in my processed foods diet, which is a good starting point. BA had a higher level of scrutiny—too strict for my current diet. Baby steps. You don't have to do it all at once. When I'm ready for scorched earth, I'll open the BA app again. Yes, winter is coming.

I found the process extremely eye-opening as far as sugar being listed as an ingredient in nearly every processed food item, including ranch dressing, BBQ sauce, and anything teriyaki. I found the sheer number of grocery items that listed sugar in their ingredients shocking. Some crackers and beef jerky products even list sugar.

More recently, I discovered it hiding in my beloved bacon. (Oh, the depravity.) I didn't even think to look until a recent BOGO sale. With bacon at nearly eight dollars for less than a pound, I found myself ready to stock up. Uncertain as to why I hadn't thought to do it sooner in my journey, I flipped the first package to read the ingredients, then the next, and so on. I must have made a guttural sound because the woman stocking meats near me asked if she could help. She pointed me to a buy-two-get-one-free brand without sugar. I took the three packages home and cooked one up for the week's breakfasts. Monday morning at the office, I bit into the first piece, shocked at the difference.

Bacon and I might be breaking up if I can't find a tasty brand. This is huge, as I've had a reputation of being one of bacon's biggest fans to the point where I've been given bacon as a present more than once. I might try a family farm online where they do everything right and order some from them.

So How Did We Get Here?

If you're not quite convinced of sugar's ill effects, like heart disease, several health gurus are screaming about the evils of sugar today. They cite a 2016 article explaining how, over fifty years ago, the sugar industry paid for a study published in 1967 that promoted fat instead of sugar as the greatest threat to our health and the cause of heart disease.[9] It's like Sugar is standing in the shadows, flashing its naked body to everybody walking by and then blaming the trench coat company when it gets caught.

But misinformation on this subject is nothing new and has been going on for nearly a century. Vinnie Tortorich, creator of the documentary *Fat*, explained how Ancel Keys, an American physiologist, blamed President Eisenhower's heart attack on the meat he ate (never mind Dwight had smoked more than three packs of unfiltered cigarettes a day for years). In the late 1950s, Keys set out to bolster his hypothesis with a six-country study, then he decided he needed a seventh and aimed to go to Crete, Greece. His conclusion stated that Greece doesn't eat meat, and they are healthy. He neglected to mention he'd purposefully delayed his arrival in Crete until Lent, when the voraciously carnivorous Greeks wouldn't eat meat for six weeks.[10] When John Yudkin of England countered the study, stating sugar was the cause of heart disease, Keys bullied the industry and had Yudkin shut down.[11]

In the 1860s, people consumed sugar only as a luxury, ingesting less than one pound per person per year. That went up greatly beginning after WWII and increasing to the modern-day average of 150 to 350 pounds of sugar eaten per person per year! One of the reasons it happened was the uptick in the consumption of processed foods. During the Great Depression, the government began paying farmers to plant or not plant certain foods, which greatly increased grain plantings, which the government then exported as

What Is *Diet?*

a commodity. That, combined with our transition from an agrarian to an industrial society in the 1940s, meant that fewer people were growing their own food.

Then, in 1969, politicians came up with Food Stamps as a way to secure votes. With this, commercial processing of foods kicked into high gear with those extra government-paid food subsidies. Later, the McGovern Committee on Food and Nutrition brought in Ancel Keys. (Yep, he's back.) They met for ten years. Normally, committees meet for days, weeks, or months, not *years*. They eventually created the modern food pyramid, promoting carbohydrates over meat, which we now know is upside-down.[12] Even the updated food pyramid continues to value carbs over protein. Carbs spike glucose just like sugar. You can probably thank the commercial farm lobby for that one.[13]

Bottom line: Make commonsense decisions. This is one of the many reasons to switch to a whole-food diet. Whole foods are single-ingredient foods: broccoli, chicken, and watermelon. These are found by shopping in the outer sections of the grocery stores, not the inner aisles with all the processed foods.

 Tip: To help break food addictions, like sugar, keep a food journal. By logging your consumption, you'll stay focused and help weed out the culprits. Give your body five to ten days to break the addiction to sugar.

What's the Solution?

A good way to start changing your diet is to learn where sugar hides in the foods you eat and make substitutions to control glucose spikes.

Hot Mess Express

On a recent trip to the Tuscany region in Italy for a writer's conference—a good excuse to travel—the group stayed at the all-inclusive Villa Febea in Chiusi, where the incomparable Alice and her staff prepared wonderful Italian dishes typical of the Tuscany region. So many conferees commented on the sheer amount of food served, usually five courses over two hours for both lunch and dinner and yet we pushed away from the table without feeling overstuffed, like back in the United States eating similar foods or at Thanksgiving.

Once home, I delved into the topic. One reason could be that Europeans generally produce a soft wheat husk with less gluten than the US counterparts, who plant a harder wheat husk variety with a high gluten content.[14] I opened my pantry to grab a box of pasta someone had gifted me months earlier after a brief conversation on ancient grains. Some of the brand's pastas are gluten-free, using brown rice instead of wheat. But this particular box contained the ancient grain einkorn. My friend had told me about it and gave me a couple of products. In return, I gifted her with Tosca Lee's novel *The Line Between*, an awesome thriller that mentions the topic of ancient grains.

On the einkorn pasta box, they had an illustration of modern wheat with einkorn wheat superimposed on top of it. Einkorn wheat is much smaller, and they claim one-fifth of the gluten, which does not give you a glucose spike. I found it in the gluten-free section of my Walmart. I stocked up and noticed I was not so full after eating a good portion of pasta made with ancient grains. I'm also not ready for a nap or starving two hours later—it satisfies hunger. Other ancient grains with low glucose spikes include spelt and emmer.

> **Tip:** Gluten-free does not mean glucose-free.

According to Jessie Inchauspé, a French biochemist and the author of *The Glucose Goddess Method* and *The Glucose Revolution*, we need glucose. Everything runs on glucose. But she warned every glucose spike shortens our life. She suggested we can "hack" our diet and reduce the glucose spikes by eating foods in order: fiber, protein and healthy fats, then carbohydrates.[15]

Start with your salad or broccoli, then eat your chicken, steak, or fish, along with avocado, walnuts, olive oil, etc. Once you've eaten your fiber and protein, then you can eat your bread, potatoes, pasta, and dessert. Jessie assures this eating order will greatly reduce or eliminate any glucose spike.

With low-glucose ancient grains, you can eat pasta without as much worry. You'll want to be careful with brown rice, chickpea, and lentil pasta. They are higher in carbohydrates than some of the other alternatives and may lead to a spike in glucose, but their protein, fiber, and nutrient content still make them a better option than traditional US wheat pasta. They're also good for avoiding gluten due to wheat allergies, wheat sensitivities, and Celiac disease. Double-check gluten-free items' ingredients. You can also substitute Konjac noodles for your oriental dishes to avoid the glucose spike.

 Tip: Studies have shown that apple cider vinegar (ACV) may lower blood glucose levels. Drink a tablespoon of apple cider vinegar (with "mother") in a glass of water before a meal to limit the glucose spike. (Caution: Do *not* use ACV if you have compromised kidneys.)

A Summary of Healthy Foods

Healthy fiber foods are good for weight loss. They lower blood sugar, fight constipation, boost heart health, and feed friendly gut bacteria. They include strawberries, avocado, broccoli, celery, and leafy greens.[16]

Protein can help minimize lean muscle loss. One study showed that women who ate ninety-two grams daily (thirty grams per meal—the size of a deck of cards) reduced their loss of function by 30 percent.[17] Protein also helps with cells, the immune system, movement, and hormones. Healthy high-protein foods include eggs, chicken breast, and cottage cheese. Greek yogurt, lean beef, turkey breast, and fish (salmon, albacore tuna, trout, halibut, and mackerel) are also very good sources of protein.[18]

For the best **healthy fats** try good cholesterol–raising, vitamin E–packed, immunity-boosting avocado—the number one fruit among keto fans. Try avocado oil, coconut oil, and extra-virgin olive oil for cooking. Fatty fish (salmon, sardines, mackerel, and anchovies) are packed with Omega-3 fatty acids—crucial to health, and your body doesn't make them. (We hit the local seafood market weekly for salmon.) Make nuts and seeds part of your regular diet for skin and brain health. Lower bad LDL cholesterol for heart health with nuts like walnuts, almonds, hazelnuts, Brazil nuts, and macadamia nuts. Flaxseeds and chia seeds are high in fiber and good fat.[19]

Other healthy fats include eggs. New science shows eggs don't raise but lower bad cholesterol. Grass-fed, organic beef is great, too, for healthy fat—if you shouldn't be eating modern wheat, then neither should your food. Medium-chain triglyceride (MCT) oil is sent to your liver and boosts your metabolism. Try it in your morning coffee, with homemade salad dressing, or baking with it instead of a third of the avocado or coconut oil you should be using instead of the usual suspects. Look for minimally processed, preferably grass-fed, full-fat dairy products, like raw milk, feta cheese, goat cheese, ricotta, and cottage cheese. You can also treat yourself to dark chocolate, as long as it is 70 percent or higher cacao for an antioxidant boost—check the baking department at the grocery store.[20]

What Is *Diet*?

Avoid processed foods and added sugar—minimize treats (yes, even the 70-percent cacao dark chocolate). Skip oils containing Omega-6 and processed foods listing them as ingredients (soybean oil, corn oil, sunflower oil, peanut oil, and sesame oil). Avoid products containing hydrogenated or partially hydrogenated oils. If they can crush or press it to get the oil, great. But if they have to process it with chemicals, don't use it.[21]

As far as cooking with oils, certain oils do bad things when heated; they oxidize and the polyunsaturated fats in these oils react chemically under heat forming free radicals (think cancer) and harmful compounds. Canola is touted as healthy, and my husband uses it in his Italian dressing made from a flavor packet, but you don't want to cook with it, as it turns toxic when heated (like an otherwise good man when drinking). Others to avoid not mentioned in the Omega-6 list above include cottonseed oil, rapeseed oil, grapeseed oil, safflower oil, and rice bran oil.[22] You can add margarine to the no-no list and skip it altogether since it's processed.

> **Tip:** If it doesn't come into your home, then you won't eat it in moments of weakness. No chips or cookies in the shopping basket, then no chips or cookies in your stomach . . . or on your belly, chin, and thighs.

Deficiencies

A word on nutritional deficiencies: many deficiencies can mimic more serious diseases.[23] For example, if you don't get enough sunlight for your body to make vitamin D3 or supplement with vitamins and you have a long-term vitamin D3 deficiency, then you could get symptoms mimicking Rheumatoid Arthritis (RA). Those symptoms include waking up sore—as if you had a workout the night before; tender feet and ankles when you first get up in the morning; stiff knees, hips, and ankles; and stiff shoulders resulting in difficulty making a tight fist. If you go to your general physician, he or she will likely misdiagnose the symptoms as RA and put you on a corticosteroid. At first, you'd get the anti-inflammatory effect, but then the corticosteroid would start eating away at your joints. Statistically, you'd be looking at a joint replacement in six years, then most people move less afterward resulting in a sedentary lifestyle, the leading cause of all mortality.

So, before you think of the worst-case scenario, ask if it could be a nutrient deficiency. It's all about how our bodies process what we put in them. Many common ailments do not come from outside in the form of diseases or pathologies. Deficiencies are happening on the inside. We need to supplement for the deficiency, which may be detected through a methylation test.[24]

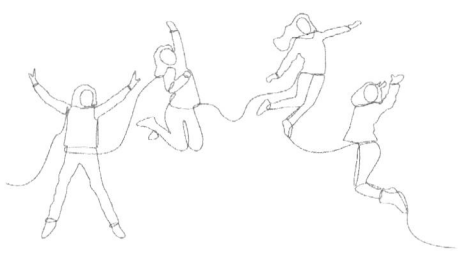

SUMMARY

If there is anything you can take away from this book, it is this: your body is having a conversation with you.

Listen to it.

You know you better than anyone else, aside from your Maker, so slow down and pay attention to what is happening (or not happening).

Take care of yourself. Allow enough time to get a full night of sleep, even if sleep doesn't come easily.

Eat right. Lay off the comfort food. Stop making a habit of fast and junk food. You don't have to be a dictator with yourself, but don't be so permissive either. Sometimes we cause more problems with our lazy diets. When the treats are daily, they are no longer treats, they're your diet. Shop the outer sections of the market (produce, dairy, meat, etc.). Real is healthier than fake or processed. Stick to whole foods—single-ingredient foods, like broccoli, eggs, fish, and cheese.

A 2021 scientific study declared, "Meat intake is positively correlated with life expectancies."[1] So don't go vegan unless you have marching orders from your doctor. It's hard enough to regain

Summary

lost muscle to boost your metabolism, especially without animal proteins.

Exercise. Start slowly and work your way up. You don't have to be a fitness guru, but you do have to move. Regularly. Walk daily. Once you've gotten used to it, try a weighted vest, resistance bands, or weights.

Ask your doctor questions about any changes in your body. Pay attention to the small things; they all add up. Keep a hot flash journal or a log for any other bothersome symptoms. Try a food journal for reactions. Show them to your doctor and be open. Share even the embarrassing things (if I can, you can). The more they know, the better they can help you. Get a hormonal baseline test now—if you haven't experienced any changes yet and are happy with how things are going—so you know your target numbers for hormones (estrogen/estradiol, progesterone, and testosterone). Remember doctors *practice* medicine. If you don't get answers or think your doctor isn't listening to you, try a new one. Opt for a specialist or a doctor of osteopathic medicine (DO) instead of an MD.

Investigate BHRT even if you don't have major hormonal change symptoms. New studies are proving the benefits if started soon after the change from perimenopause to menopause, and they're disproving many cancer-related assumptions. Dig deep and pound on doors to find the answer to what's best for you—we're all different.

Present your concerns to your Maker. He created you. He knows you. He knows what's right with you; He knows what's wrong with you. Ask Him for insights. Ask Him for wisdom for you and your doctor. But above all else, sit at His feet and let Him love on you. Let Him give you patience for your oh-so-common condition that seems to affect every woman differently. Give Him your frustrations and let Him exchange your ashes for beauty. He will give you the grace to endure these years.

Summary

You are not alone in this. So many of us are hit hard with changing hormones. Does misery love company? I wouldn't wish this on anyone, but it does bring me a certain amount of comfort knowing it's not just me this is happening to. Though my journey is decidedly atypical and next to nothing worked for me, everything I tried did work for most others.

In the documentary *The Longevity Film*, the host, Kale Brock, visited three of the five known Blue Zones, communities where the average life expectancy is ten to fifteen years more than what we experience on average in America.[2] They have more centenarians clustered in these five communities than anywhere else in the world. Brock set out to find out why. I'm not usually keen on documentaries, preferring action movies instead, but *Longevity* entertained me enough with gorgeous views of these areas and engaging interactions with the locals.

I mention *Longevity* because I think the main premise of living well hits home as a common thread throughout this book's chapters. According to the movie, these people don't just live longer but enjoy healthier longer lives. They don't know the lifestyle of prescriptions. These communities shared certain aspects.

Food: They eat natural, seasonal foods they grow at home or purchase at locally grown markets. These foods are low in calories and high in nutrients, like seaweed, veggies, and fish in the Okinawa, Japan, community. They eat only vegetables in the Seventh-Day Adventist community of Loma Linda, California. And in Ikaria, Greece, they consume fish and veggies, with red meat only eaten once per week, but all food in moderation. All of these populations are near the ocean, so I think the fish rich in Omega-3 fatty acids is key. Salmon is my favorite. My husband gets ours from a local fish market, caught fresh. If you routinely get the nutrition right, then you don't have to hit the target every time.[3]

Summary

Exercise: People in these Blue Zone areas move their bodies regularly in exercise three to five hours per week. The more you move the more you can move. Movement is life.[4]

Happiness: They are happy. Being happy releases chemicals in the brain. Things that make you feel happy make you live longer. Get together with your friends for conversation and a good meal. Isolation is death.[5]

Relationships: Cultivate good family and friend relationships. Live with at least one other person who loves and cares for you and whom you care for. Enjoy multigenerational relationships with your grandchildren or other young ones (exercise together, dance, or play on the floor together with their toys). You'll stay younger in mind.[6]

Live in the moment: These people seem to be a real community. When they get together, which is often, they aren't on their phones. Social media does not equate to relationships.[7]

That last one is big—live in the moment. I have a dear cousin who, with her husband and daughter, all got the same tattoo: be here now. I'm not crazy about tattoos, but I appreciate the sentiments. I recently ate a "fun" pack of peanut M&M's and got busy while I ate the last three. The enjoyment was much less than it had been with the others. The enjoyment of those last three would have been the same if I'd swallowed them with water like a pill. I could've pushed back from the keyboard for thirty seconds to enjoy them all, but I didn't. If you're going to eat a treat once in a while, make it worth it by enjoying it. Be in the moment.

Multitasking will suck the life right out of you. Do it when you have to beat a deadline, but when you can slow down for a little bit, do it. Savor the treats. Enjoy the relationships. Take a deep breath and exhale slowly. Do what makes you happy (as long as it's legal and moral), and take care of yourself.

Summary

Lately, some experts are doubting the conclusions made by others regarding the Blue Zones. Gary Brecka said he thinks it has less to do with lifestyle and more to do with the fact that these Blue Zones are closer to the equator and those populations are getting more sunlight. Supplement with Vitamin D3 if you're not getting enough sunlight.[8]

You're coming into the best years of your life. There are several reasons to look forward to menopause. You can say goodbye to periods and the associated PMS, which can include severe headaches. The uterine fibroids you can get during pregnancies or perimenopause should shrink. Those who've had children may see menopause as a time to shift from parent to grandparent. You can focus on taking care of yourself. It's also a time to take stock in life and a time you can ease into the well-earned confidence and wisdom.[9]

So, hang in there.

Dean relayed the thoughts of his brother-in-law who warned that once you get to a certain age, you disappear from society. One day the younger people just stop noticing you. You're no longer considered attractive or "hot," you are now "attractive for your age." People dismiss you if they notice you at all.

Yikes.

My husband swears this just happened to us at the mall when a security guard ignored us when Dean tried to get attention as the young man walked by. But since I aim to go down swinging, I like the study showing how older people feel better about themselves. Self-esteem is at an all-time high at the age of sixty and can remain high for a decade.[10]

Although it can be tough, and tougher on some of us than others, this is not the end of the world. You can get through this. Commiserate with your fellow travelers on this road and be honest and open with your doctor. One young doctor on Instagram bemoaned the fact that she had only five hours of total instruction during med

Summary

school about women's health regarding menopause and women's aging. Be patient with your doctor; you might have to learn together. But don't walk away satisfied with no answers or a one-size-fits-all plan while you continue to suffer.

You might be crowning the hill and starting down the backside, but for many, the grass is greener on this side. Even with the bevy of symptoms I've dealt with, I like much about being over the hill and careening down the other side. In many ways, it's a lot easier than my youthful years. Mostly because I've stopped making so many detrimental, stupid choices in life.

After a decade of perimenopause behind me, I am now face to face with menopause. I'm both disheartened and encouraged to know extreme cases only last seven to twelve years. My hot flashes are ebbing and flowing, occasionally occurring daily (and nightly), even with bioidentical hormones. But I'm starting to see larger swaths of "deep sleep" on my fitness watch, which monitors sleep levels. I choose to believe this too shall pass—kicking and screaming but nonetheless pass. Be good to yourself in all ways. Now and later.

I wish you well on your journey to hormonal freedom.

Mr. Spock said, "Live long and prosper," which actor Leonard Nimoy first coined based on a Jewish greeting.[11]

Jesus spoke peace over us and said by his stripes we are healed. Learn to walk in that healing enacted two millennia ago.

Pray you are miraculously delivered from your symptoms. God says you have not because you ask not. But if your healing does not immediately manifest, as mine did not, I wish you peace of mind and wisdom in knowing what is in your power to lessen your symptoms.

Be proactive.

Be consistent.

I hope we all learn how to live better.

Life is too short to let menopause symptoms get the best of us.

ACKNOWLEDGMENTS

Tina Yeager stared past my self-doubts and into my soul, suggesting one year at the Florida Christian Writers Conference that I take all my whining about menopause and put it in a book with my humor. Without her, I would have continued in my exciting world of creative fiction writing. Instead, I entered the world of mind-numbing citations and sourcing—good times.

Thank you to my friend and editor, Jan Powell, who encouraged me from the beginning of my writing journey, without whom I would have quit writing that first year. I am in awe of Susan Cornell, whose edits at the publishing company (Iron Stream Media) made this book so much better. I am grateful to Irene Wintermeyer, Sefi Adkins, and the other critique group members at Word Weavers International—Brevard County and Orlando chapters. They endured my menopause manuscript while others brought fun samples of their writing. Nevertheless, the group graciously gave excellent feedback each month.

Many thanks to Del Duduit, my first agent at C.Y.L.E. literary agency, who scooped me up when Bethany Jett told him how compliant I'd been under her coaching. I appreciate my current agent extraordinaire, Andy Clapp, who kept me on when he inherited Del's clients—I know he didn't keep them all. Andy knocked on many doors and revisited publishers enough to land me a contract for this book. And thanks to John Herring at Iron Stream Media for taking a chance on me. How are those grandkids?

I am eternally thankful to Rhonda Bray, who first clued me in that menopause, my great nemesis, was the name of my pain. Many thanks to my friends, like Barbara Crotteau, who encouraged me,

Acknowledgments

and friends who spoke words of Life over me from Freedom Christian Center in Viera, like Erica Ross and Lue Ann Grosdidier.

 This book's existence is in no way due to the efforts of my fourth-grade teacher at Fort Knox Elementary School, who moved me into the smart kids' group and then, within the hour, moved me back out. It is partly due to my Park Avenue Baptist Church Singles group friend Dave Bush, who went online and took an IQ test, proving that I'm smarter than a NASA engineer, if only by one point. Thank you, Dave; it made me feel smart for the first time. That boost enabled me to finish my BS degree and eventually start writing.

 This book came out of great suffering and compassion for those who walk this crazy, long road so that your suffering may not be as bad as mine—light in the darkness; you are not alone. I pray your mind, body, marriage, and other relationships survive this wild ride.

NOTES

3. What Are We Talking About?

1. "Postmenopause," Cleveland Clinic, accessed March 15, 2021, https://my.clevelandclinic.org/health/diseases/21837-postmenopause.
2. "Reproductive Hormones," Endocrine Society, January 24, 2022, https://www.endocrine.org/patient-engagement/endocrine-library/hormones-and-endocrine-function/reproductive-hormones.
3. Kati Forholt, APRN, "Sally Friscea Visit Summary," July 28, 2022.
4. Forholt, "Sally Friscea Visit Summary."
5. Christiane Northrup, MD, "Nutrition: Hormone-Balancing Food Plan," Christiane Northrup MD, accessed August 9, 2023, https://www.drnorthrup.com/nutrition-hormone-balancing-food-plan/.
6. "Does Caffeine Make Menopause Symptoms Worse?," Penn Medicine, Lancaster General Health, August 1, 2016, https://www.lancastergeneralhealth.org/health-hub-home/2016/august/menopause--caffeine--hot-flashes.

4. Insomnia

1. Michael L. Perlis et al., *Cognitive Behavioral Treatment of Insomnia: A Session-by-Session Guide* (New York: Springer, 2008).
2. Charles M. Morin et al., "The Insomnia Severity Index: Psychometric Indicators to Detect Insomnia Cases and Evaluate Treatment Response," National Library of Medicine, National Center for Biotechnology Information, National Institutes of Health, May 1, 2011, https://www.ncbi.nlm.nih.gov/pmc/articles/PMC3079939.
3. Perlis et al., *Cognitive Behavioral Treatment of Insomnia*, 18.
4. Howard LeWine, MD, "Does Exercising at Night Affect Sleep?," Harvard Health Publishing, Harvard Medical School, April 1, 2019, https://www.health.harvard.edu/staying-healthy/does-exercising-at-night-affect-sleep.
5. Some of the technical information on natural remedies was taken from WebMD. Debra Fulghum Bruce, PhD, "Natural Sleep Aids

and Remedies," WebMD, January 26, 2022, https://www.webmd.com/women/natural-sleep-remedies#2.
6. Michael Downey, "Beyond Depression . . . SAMe Broad-Spectrum Protection Against Disorders of Aging," Life Extension, August 2023, https://www.lifeextension.com/magazine/2014/4/beyond-depression-same-broad-spectrum-protection-against-disorders-of-aging.
7. "S-adenosylmethionine," Mount Sinai Health System, accessed March 8, 2024, https://www.mountsinai.org/health-library/supplement/s-adenosylmethionine.

5. Hormonal Rage and Mood Swings

1. Danielle Dresden, "What Causes Mood Swings During Menopause?," Medical News Today, May 22, 2017. Accessed on July 22, 2024, from the Internet Archive, https://web.archive.org/web/20201001163446/https://www.medicalnewstoday.com/articles/317566#Overview.

6. Hot Flashes and Night Sweats

1. This list is from "Hot Flashes," Mayo Clinic, December 12, 2023, https://www.mayoclinic.org/diseases-conditions/hot-flashes/symptoms-causes/syc-20352790.
2. "Hot Flashes," Mayo Clinic.
3. Rachel Jacoby Zoldan, "The Embr Wave Bracelet Claims to Regulate Your Body Temperature—Does It Work?," *USA Today*, February 21, 2019, https://reviewed.usatoday.com/home-outdoors/features/embr-wave-review.
4. Marie Suszynski, "Menopause and Sweating," WebMD, July 20, 2011, https://www.webmd.com/menopause/features/menopause-sweating-11#1.
5. Suszynski, "Menopause and Sweating."
6. Suszynski, "Menopause and Sweating."
7. Joana Cavaco Silva, "Coping With Menopausal Hot Flashes and Night Sweats," July 21, 2023, https://www.medicalnewstoday.com/articles/322351.
8. "Coping With Menopausal Hot Flashes and Night Sweats."

Notes

7. Hair

1. Nadeem Badshah, "Scientists May Have Discovered Why Hair Turns Grey," *The Guardian*, April 19, 2023, https://www.theguardian.com/science/2023/apr/19/scientists-may-have-discovered-why-hair-turns-grey.
2. "Why Lime-Yellow Fire Trucks Are Safer Than Red," American Psychological Association, 2014, https://www.apa.org/topics/safety-design/fire-engine-color-safety.

8. Skin

1. "Vaginal Atrophy (Atrophic Vaginitis)," Harvard Health Publishing, Harvard Medical School, February 12, 2024, https://www.health.harvard.edu/a_to_z/vaginal-atrophy-atrophic-vaginitis-a-to-z.
2. "Vaginal Atrophy," Mayo Clinic, September 17, 2021, https://www.mayoclinic.org/diseases-conditions/vaginal-atrophy/symptoms-causes/syc-20352288.
3. Mandy Ferreira, "Causes of and Treatments for Crepey Skin," Healthline, February 21, 2023, https://www.healthline.com/health/crepey-skin.
4. Mili Godio, "11 Best Treatments for Dry, Cracked Heels, According to Dermatologists," NBC Select, November 14, 2019, https://www.nbcnews.com/better/lifestyle/how-care-dry-cracked-heels-according-dermatologists-ncna1080001.
5. Godio, "11 Best Treatments."
6. Godio, "11 Best Treatments."
7. Godio, "11 Best Treatments."
8. Shannon Johnson, "Varicose Vein Stripping," Healthline, June 15, 2021, https://www.healthline.com/health/varicose-vein-stripping.
9. "Easy Bruising: Why Does It Happen?," Mayo Clinic, September 20, 2023, https://www.mayoclinic.org/healthy-lifestyle/healthy-aging/in-depth/easy-bruising/art-20045762.
10. "Skin Cancer Early Detection," Fred Hutch Cancer Center, accessed March 30, 2021, https://www.seattlecca.org/prevention/skin-cancer-early-detection.
11. "Skin Cancer Early Detection," Fred Hutch Cancer Center.
12. "Skin Cancer Early Detection," Fred Hutch Cancer Center.

Notes

13. "Five or More Blistering Sunburns Before Age 20 May Increase Melanoma Risk by 80 Percent," American Association for Cancer Research, May 29, 2014, https://aacrnews.wordpress.com/2014/05/29/five-or-more-blistering-sunburns-before-age-20-may-increase-melanoma-risk-by-80-percent/.
14. "Efudex Cream—Uses, Side Effects, and More," n.d. (accessed March 20, 2021), https://www.webmd.com/drugs/2/drug-3723/efudex-topical/details.
15. "Age Spots (Liver Spots)," Mayo Clinic, February 11, 2022, https://www.mayoclinic.org/diseases-conditions/age-spots/symptoms-causes/syc-20355859.
16. "Do Retinoids Really Reduce Wrinkles?," Harvard Health Publishing, Harvard Medical School, March 3, 2022, https://www.health.harvard.edu/staying-healthy/do-retinoids-really-reduce-wrinkles.
17. Lana Burgess, "What Are the Best Ways to Get Rid of Large Pores?," Medical News Today, April 18, 2023, https://www.medicalnewstoday.com/articles/320775.
18. Zawn Villines, "Why Are Some People Ticklish?," Medical News Today, July 20, 2023, https://www.medicalnewstoday.com/articles/322100.

9. Nails

1. Corey Whelan, "How Can I Treat Hangnails?," Healthline, March 8, 2019, https://www.healthline.com/health/how-to-get-rid-of-hangnails.
2. Jon Johnson, "All You Need to Know About Ridges in Fingernails," Medical News Today, November 30, 2023, https://www.medicalnewstoday.com/articles/319867.

10. Eyes

1. Jane Chertoff, "How to Read Your Eye Prescription," Healthline, July 18, 2024, https://www.healthline.com/health/eye-health/how-bad-is-my-eye-prescription.
2. Doctor Eye Health, "Contact Lenses for Beginners | How to Put in Contacts," August 27, 2019, https://www.youtube.com/watch?v=wlPyYkq3LnY.
3. *Merriam-Webster Dictionary*, s.v. "presbyopia," accessed April 11, 2024, https://www.merriam-webster.com/dictionary/presbyopia.

Notes

4. "Cataracts," Mayo Clinic, September 28, 2023, https://www.mayoclinic.org/diseases-conditions/cataracts/symptoms-causes/syc-20353790.
5. "Is the Degradation of Depth Perception an Inevitable Result of Aging?," American Academy of Ophthalmology, February 21, 2014, https://www.aao.org/eye-health/ask-ophthalmologist-q/is-degradation-of-depth-perception-inevitable-resu.
6. "Can LASIK Improve Depth Perception," Peña Eye Institute, June 22, 2017, https://www.penaeye.com/blog/2017/06/22/can-lasik-improve-depth-perception-184003.
7. Kun Hwang, MD, PhD, Dae Joong Kim, PhD, and Seong Kee Kim, MD, "Does the Upper Eyelid Skin Become Thinner With Age?," *Journal of Craniofacial Surgery* 17, no. 3 (May 2006): 474–76, accessed March 30, 2021, https://journals.lww.com/jcraniofacialsurgery/Abstract/2006/05000/Does_the_Upper_Eyelid_Skin_Become_Thinner_With.14.aspx.
8. "Why You Should Be Using a Sleep Mask Every Single Night," *Shape*, October 4, 2022, https://www.shape.com/lifestyle/mind-and-body/sleep-mask-benefits.
9. "Why You Should Be Using a Sleep Mask Every Single Night."
10. "The Aging Eye: When to Worry About Eyelid Problems," Harvard Health Publishing, Harvard Medical School, October 10, 2019, https://www.health.harvard.edu/staying-healthy/the-aging-eye-when-to-worry-about-eyelid-problems.

11. Inner Ear

1. "Aging Changes in the Senses" NIH National Library of Medicine, MedlinePlus, accessed March 20, 2021, https://medlineplus.gov/ency/article/004013.htm.
2. Eleni Xenos, "10 Tips to Beat Motion Sickness," Amazon One Medical, November 1, 2018, https://www.onemedical.com/blog/get-well/motion-sickness-cures.
3. Xenos, "10 Tips to Beat Motion Sickness."
4. "Home Remedies for Vertigo," WebMD, June 6, 2023, https://www.webmd.com/brain/home-remedies-vertigo#1.
5. Eileen Durward, "Does Menopause Affect Your Ears?," A.Vogel, July 19, 2021, https://www.avogel.co.uk/health/menopause/videos/does-menopause-affect-your-ears/.

Notes

6. Kevin St. Clergy, "Excessive Ear Wax: Common Culprits," Helping Me Hear, July 29, 2022, https://www.helpingmehear.com/hearing-loss-articles/excessive-ear-wax-common-culprits/.

12. Mouth

1. Douglas Main, "5 Surprising Ways to Banish Bad Breath," Livescience.com, September 30, 2013, https://www.livescience.com/40052-get-rid-bad-breath.html.
2. "Healthier Options for Mouthwash," Guzaitis Dental Group (blog), https://gdgdental.com/healthier-options-for-mouthwash-are-out-there/.
3. Lauren Janowiecki, "6 All-Natural Mouthwashes to Help Break Your Listerine Habit," Thomas C. Volck, DDS, Todd Busdiecker, DDS (blog), https://www.drthomasvolck.com/post/6-all-natural-mouthwashes-to-help-break-your-listerine-habit.
4. Max Lugavere, "Nitric Oxide: The Holy Grail of Inflammation & Disease - Fix This for Longevity | Dr. Nathan Bryan," September 20, 2023, https://www.youtube.com/watch?v=qGVLqLxAl0I.
5. "Throw Away the Tums! Healthy Alternatives to Antacids," Boston Functional Nutrition, accessed October 9, 2023, https://bostonfunctionalnutrition.com/throw-away-the-tums-healthy-alternatives-to-antacids/.
6. "Understanding Canker Sores—the Basics," WebMD, September 6, 2023, https://www.webmd.com/oral-health/understanding-canker-sores-basics.
7. "Choking: First Aid," Mayo Clinic, https://www.mayoclinic.org/first-aid/first-aid-choking/basics/art-20056637.
8. Julie A. Y. Chichero, "Age-Related Changes to Eating and Swallowing Impact Frailty: Aspiration, Choking Risk, Modified Food Texture and Autonomy of Choice," National Library of Medicine, National Center for Biotechnology Information, National Institutes of Health, October 12, 2018, accessed March 30, 2021, https://www.ncbi.nlm.nih.gov/pmc/articles/PMC6371116/.
9. Erica Smalley, BS, LVN, "Hard to Swallow: When Seniors Experience Chronic Choking; Part 1 of a 4-Part Series for Family Caregivers," A Hand to Hold. Accessed on July 24, 2024, from the Internet Archive, https://web.archive.org/web/20200118004447/http://www.ahandtoholdsd.com/hard-to-swallow-when-seniors-experience-chronic-choking/.

Notes

10. "Swallowing Exercises: How to Do Tongue-Strengthening Exercises," Johns Hopkins Medicine, November 19, 2019, https://www.hopkinsmedicine.org/health/treatment-tests-and-therapies/swallowing-exercises-how-to-do-tonguestrengthening-exercises.
11. "Swallowing Exercises: How to Do Tongue-Strengthening Exercises," Johns Hopkins Medicine.

13. Nose

1. "Snoring," Mayo Clinic, December 22, 2017, https://www.mayoclinic.org/diseases-conditions/snoring/symptoms-causes/syc-20377694.
2. "Snoring."
3. "Snoring."
4. "Snoring."
5. Tamara Newell, "Deviated Septum: What Does It Mean?," WebMD, October 4, 2023, https://www.webmd.com/allergies/deviated-septum#1.
6. Andrea Markowitz, "Getting Worse With Age," *Chicago Tribune*, May 13, 2019, https://www.chicagotribune.com/lifestyles/ct-xpm-2010-07-23-sc-health-0723-allergies-seniors-20100723-story.html.
7. Jacquelyn Cafasso, "How to Do a Sinus Flush at Home," January 28, 2019, Healthline, https://www.healthline.com/health/sinus-flush.
8. Stephanie Watson, "Migraines and Menopause," WebMD, February 2, 2022, https://www.webmd.com/migraines-headaches/migraines-menopause.
9. Watson, "Migraines and Menopause."
10. Watson, "Migraines and Menopause."

14. Muscle Tone

1. Katherine Scoleri CPT, "Core Stabilizing Ab Exercises to Help Prevent Injury in Seniors," Healthline, October 3, 2019, https://www.healthline.com/health/senior-health/ab-exercises.
2. "Want a Stronger Core? Skip the Sit-ups," Harvard Health Publishing, Harvard Medical School, May 23, 2023, https://www.health.harvard.edu/staying-healthy/want-a-stronger-core-skip-the-sit-ups.
3. Hilary Brueck, "Fitness Experts Agree That Sit-Ups Are Worthless—Here Are 9 Moves They Recommend Instead," *Business Insider*,

Notes

July 15, 2018, https://www.businessinsider.com/fitness-experts-sit-ups-worthless-what-to-do-instead-2018-7.

4. "Working Out When You're Over 50," WebMD, accessed March 30, 2021, https://www.webmd.com/fitness-exercise/ss/slideshow-exercise-after-age-50.

5. Peter Crosta, "Everything You Need to Know About Cellulite," Medical News Today, November 13, 2023, https://www.medicalnewstoday.com/articles/149465.

6. Dr. Eric Berg, DC, "Get Rid of Cellulite for Good: Dr. Berg's Better Way to Lose Flabby Fat," January 3, 2022, https://www.youtube.com/watch?v=0lCuHaDj5pg.

7. Dr. Mike Roussell, "Ask The Diet Doctor: Does the Food Combining Diet Work?," *Shape*, December 3, 2012. Accessed on July 25, 2024, from the Internet Archive, https://web.archive.org/web/20210925213804/https://www.shape.com/healthy-eating/diet-tips/ask-diet-doctor-does-food-combining-diet-work.

8. Crosta, "Everything You Need to Know About Cellulite."

9. Crosta, "Everything You Need to Know About Cellulite."

10. Berg, "Get Rid of Cellulite for Good."

11. Berg, "Get Rid of Cellulite for Good."

12. Berg, "Get Rid of Cellulite for Good."

13. "Strength Training: Get Stronger, Leaner, Healthier," Mayo Clinic, April 29, 2023, https://www.mayoclinic.org/healthy-lifestyle/fitness/in-depth/strength-training/art-20046670.

14. Stephanie Mansour, "Low Weight High Reps vs. High Weight Low Reps: What's the Best Way to Strength Train?," *Today*, March 16, 2022, https://www.today.com/health/diet-fitness/low-weight-high-reps-or-high-weight-low-reps-rcna20248.

15. Berg, "Get Rid of Cellulite for Good."

16. Crosta, "Everything You Need to Know About Cellulite."

17. "The Importance of Stretching," Harvard Health Publishing, Harvard Medical School, March 14, 2022, https://www.health.harvard.edu/staying-healthy/the-importance-of-stretching.

18. "Bra Fit Tips & Tests," Her Room, accessed March 30, 2021, https://www.herroom.com/bra-fitting,902,30.html.

Notes

19. "Breast Pain: 10 Reasons Your Breasts May Hurt," Johns Hopkins Medicine, November 1, 2022, https://www.hopkinsmedicine.org/health/conditions-and-diseases/breast-pain-10-reasons-your-breasts-may-hurt.
20. "Breast Pain," Johns Hopkins.
21. Catherine Renton, "Symptoms of Breast Pain in Menopause," Very Well Health, May 17, 2021. Accessed on July 26, 2024, from the Internet Archive, https://web.archive.org/web/20210618021455/https://www.verywellhealth.com/breast-pain-in-menopause-symptoms-5180788.
22. "Aging Changes in the Kidneys and Bladder," NIH National Library of Medicine, MedlinePlus, accessed March 31, 2021, https://medlineplus.gov/ency/article/004010.htm.
23. Kathryn Watson and Adrienne Santos-Longhurst, "7 Urinary Tract Infection (UTI) Treatments at Home," Healthline, June 24, 2024, https://www.healthline.com/nutrition/uti-home-remedies.
24. Katherine Lee, "9 Smart Ways to Manage a Leaky Bladder," Everyday Health, May 27, 2023, https://www.everydayhealth.com/incontinence/kegel-exercises-for-urinary-incontinence.aspx.
25. James Woods, MD, and Elizabeth Warner, MD, "Spice, Pickles for Leg Cramps . . . Can It Be That Simple?," University of Rochester Medical Center, November 15, 2016, https://www.urmc.rochester.edu/ob-gyn/ur-medicine-menopause-and-womens-health/menopause-blog/november-2016-1/spice-pickles-for-leg-cramps-can-it-be-that-simple.aspx.
26. Peter M. Tiidus, Dawn A. Lowe, and Marybeth Brown, "Estrogen Replacement and Skeletal Muscle: Mechanisms and Population Health," National Institutes of Health, National Library of Medicine, National Center for Biotechnology Information, July 18, 2013, https://www.ncbi.nlm.nih.gov/pmc/articles/PMC5504400/.
27. Team MM, "What To Do About Muscle Spasms?," Megs Menopause, February 18, 2020. Accessed July 26, 2024, from the Internet Archive, https://web.archive.org/web/20200225181426/https://megsmenopause.com/2020/02/18/muscle-spasm/.
28. Woods and Warner, "Spice, Pickles for Leg Cramps . . . Can It Be That Simple?"

Notes

29. "Restless Legs Syndrome," Mayo Clinic, January 26, 2024, https://www.mayoclinic.org/diseases-conditions/restless-legs-syndrome/symptoms-causes/syc-20377168.

15. Metabolism and Weight Gain

1. *Merriam-Webster Dictionary*, s.v. "muffin top," https://www.merriam-webster.com/dictionary/muffin%20top.
2. Julia Dellitt, "How Is Metabolism Different in Men and Women?," *Aaptiv* (blog), June 20, 2019, https://aaptiv.com/magazine/male-metabolism-common-questions.
3. Dellitt, "How Is Metabolism Different in Men and Women?"
4. Charles Patrick Davis MD, PhD, "Definition of Metabolism," RxList, accessed April 12, 2024, https://www.rxlist.com/metabolism/definition.htm.
5. Bowling Green State University, "New Research Shows Benefit of Interval Training for Women," ScienceDaily, August 27, 2013, www.sciencedaily.com/releases/2013/08/130827111919.htm.
6. "How to Build Lean Muscle After 50," *Prime Women* (blog), April 29, 2023, https://primewomen.com/health/fitness/you-can-build-lean-muscle-after-50/.
7. "How to Build Lean Muscle After 50," *Prime Women* (blog).
8. Jane Chertoff, "What Are the Benefits of Walking?," Healthline, November 8, 2018, https://www.healthline.com/health/benefits-of-walking#immunity.
9. "How to Build Lean Muscle After 50," *Prime Women* (blog).
10. Erin Donnelly Michos, MD, MHS, "Why Cholesterol Matters for Women," Johns Hopkins Medicine. Accessed on July 29, 2024, from the Internet Archive, https://web.archive.org/web/20220117203937/https://www.hopkinsmedicine.org/health/wellness-and-prevention/why-cholesterol-matters-for-women.
11. Michos, "Why Cholesterol Matters for Women."
12. Łukasz Białek and Bogna Szyk, "Cholesterol Ratio Calculator," Omni Calculator, January 18, 2024, https://www.omnicalculator.com/health/cholesterol-ratio.
13. Michos, "Why Cholesterol Matters for Women."

Notes

14. Dr. Josh Axe, DC, DNM, CN, "Einkorn Flour: The Superior Ancient Grain Compared to Whole Wheat," Dr. Axe, November 19, 2023, https://draxe.com/nutrition/einkorn-flour/.

16. Digestive Issues

1. Julie Wilkinson BSN, RN, "Can Excessive Gas Be a Sign of a Medical Problem?," Verywell Health, April 9, 2024, https://www.verywellhealth.com/when-should-i-worry-about-passing-too-much-gas-796838.
2. "Why Do I Keep Farting?," Cleveland Clinic, October 14, 2022, https://health.clevelandclinic.org/what-causes-flatulence-and-what-to-do-when-its-a-problem-for-you/.
3. Marjorie Hecht, "Immediate Relief for Trapped Gas: 9 Home Remedies and Prevention Tips," Healthline, January 24, 2024, https://www.healthline.com/health/immediate-relief-for-trapped-gas-home-remedies-and-prevention-tips.
4. Wilkinson, "Can Excessive Gas Be a Sign of a Medical Problem?"
5. Cynthia Weiss, "Mayo Clinic Q and A: Increasing Fiber Intake for Constipation Relief," Mayo Clinic News Network, August 10, 2021, https://newsnetwork.mayoclinic.org/discussion/mayo-clinic-q-and-a-increasing-fiber-intake-for-constipation-relief/.
6. Weiss, "Mayo Clinic Q and A: Increasing Fiber Intake for Constipation Relief."
7. "Why Do I Keep Farting?," Cleveland Clinic.
8. Sue Stetzel, "Degassing Beans: Here's How to Silence the 'Musical Fruit,'" *Taste of Home*, March 8, 2021, https://www.tasteofhome.com/article/degassing-beans/.
9. Kelli McGrane MS RD, "How to Cook Beans to Reduce Gas," Foodal, August 11, 2020, https://foodal.com/knowledge/how-to/cook-beans-reduce-gas/.
10. "Why Do I Keep Farting?," Cleveland Clinic.
11. "Chart of High-Fiber Foods," Mayo Clinic, November 23, 2023, https://www.mayoclinic.org/healthy-lifestyle/nutrition-and-healthy-eating/in-depth/high-fiber-foods/art-20050948.
12. Sharon O'Brien MS, PGDip, "Top 20 Foods High in Soluble Fiber," Healthline, January 11, 2024, https://www.healthline.com/nutrition/foods-high-in-soluble-fiber.

Notes

13. WebMD Editorial Contributors, "Worst Foods High in Lectins," WebMD, November 10, 2022, https://www.webmd.com/diet/foods-high-in-lectins#1.
14. Remy Tennant, "6 Natural Lectin Blockers (and How to Get More of Them)," Human Food Bar, January 18, 2023, https://humanfoodbar.com/lectin-free-diet/lectin-blocker/.
15. "Why Do I Keep Farting?," Cleveland Clinic.
16. Eric Lyday, "What's Your Poop Telling You?," Daily Infographic, July 19, 2014, https://www.dailyinfographic.com/whats-your-poop-telling-you-infographic.

17. Joints

1. Peter H. Gott, MD, "What's the Difference Between Bursitis and Arthritis?," *The Spokesman-Review* (Spokane, WA), September 30, 2008, https://www.spokesman.com/stories/2008/sep/30/whats-the-difference-between-bursitis-and/.
2. Gott, "What's the Difference Between Bursitis and Arthritis?"
3. Gott, "What's the Difference Between Bursitis and Arthritis?"
4. Matthew Ezerioha, MD, "Let's Dig Into Everything About RA," Rheumatoid Arthritis, Rheumatoid Arthritis Support Network, September 13, 2018, https://www.rheumatoidarthritis.org/ra/.
5. Ezerioha, "Let's Dig Into Everything About RA."
6. Ezerioha, "Let's Dig Into Everything About RA."
7. Ezerioha, "Let's Dig Into Everything About RA."
8. "Cortisone Shots," Mayo Clinic, September 21, 2023, https://www.mayoclinic.org/tests-procedures/cortisone-shots/about/pac-20384794.
9. "Weather and Arthritis Pain," Arthritis Foundation. Accessed on August 7, 2024, from the Internet Archive, https://web.archive.org/web/20210202225942/http://blog.arthritis.org/living-with-arthritis/weather-arthritis-pain/.
10. "Will Joint Cracking Cause Osteoarthritis?," WebMD, March 2, 2023, https://www.webmd.com/osteoarthritis/joint-cracking-osteoarthritis.
11. "Dupuytren Contracture," Mayo Clinic, September 28, 2023, https://www.mayoclinic.org/diseases-conditions/dupuytrens-contracture/diagnosis-treatment/drc-20371949.

Notes

12. Paolo Juden, "Frozen Shoulder: Menopause Increases the Risk | Here's Why, Treatments, and More" Shoulder Savvy, March 21, 2022, https://shouldersavvy.com/frozen-shoulder-menopause/.
13. Amberley Davis, "How to Ease Joint Pain During the Menopause," Patient, April 1, 2022, https://patient.info/news-and-features/how-to-ease-joint-pain-during-the-menopause.
14. Helen Millar, "The Link Between Frozen Shoulder and Menopause," Medical News Today, January 20, 2022, https://www.medicalnewstoday.com/articles/frozen-shoulder-menopause#treatment.
15. Millar, "The Link Between Frozen Shoulder and Menopause."

18. Bones

1. "DEXA Bone Density Scans," Riverview Health, Healthlines, May 12, 2022, https://riverview.org/blog/orthopedics/bone-health-for-aging-women/.
2. "Osteopenia," Cleveland Clinic, n.d. (accessed December 2, 2021), https://my.clevelandclinic.org/health/diseases/21855-osteopenia.
3. Caitlin Geng, "How Does Estrogen Affect Osteoporosis?," September 20, 2023, https://www.medicalnewstoday.com/articles/estrogen-and-osteoporosis.
4. "Osteoporosis Treatment: Medications Can Help," Mayo Clinic, November 1, 2023, https://www.mayoclinic.org/diseases-conditions/osteoporosis/in-depth/osteoporosis-treatment/art-20046869.
5. "Osteoporosis Treatment: Medications Can Help," Mayo Clinic.
6. Katarzyna Maresz, "Proper Calcium Use: Vitamin K2 as a Promoter of Bone and Cardiovascular Health," National Institutes of Health, National Library of Medicine, National Center for Biotechnology Information, February 2015, https://www.ncbi.nlm.nih.gov/pmc/articles/PMC4566462/.
7. "Calcium Supplements: Should You Take Them?," Johns Hopkins Medicine, November 1, 2022, https://www.hopkinsmedicine.org/health/wellness-and-prevention/calcium-supplements-should-you-take-them.
8. Kerri-Ann Jennings, MS RD, and Rachael Ajmera, MS, RD, "Top 15 Calcium-Rich Foods (Many Are Nondairy)," Healthline, December 8, 2023, https://www.healthline.com/nutrition/15-calcium-rich-foods.

Notes

9. "Osteoporosis," National Institutes of Health, National Institute on Aging, accessed May 19, 2021, https://www.nia.nih.gov/health/osteoporosis.
10. "Aging Changes in the Bones - Muscles - Joints," National Institutes of Health National Library of Medicine, MedlinePlus, July 21, 2022, https://medlineplus.gov/ency/article/004015.htm.

19. Healing

1. Erin Beresini, "Why Does Healing Take Longer as I Age?," Outside, May 16, 2013 (updated February 24, 2022), https://www.outsideonline.com/1784116/why-does-healing-take-longer-i-age.
2. Beresini, "Why Does Healing Take Longer as I Age?"
3. Eric Nagourney, "Why Am I Still on Crutches?," *New York Times*, October 24, 2012, https://www.nytimes.com/2012/10/25/booming/baby-boomer-injuries-heal-more-slowly.html.
4. Nagourney, "Why Am I Still on Crutches?"
5. "Age And Its Effect on Wound Healing," Advanced Tissue, November 6, 2014. Accessed on August 8, 2024, from the Internet Archive, https://web.archive.org/web/20210502000657/https://advancedtissue.com/2014/11/age-effect-wound-healing/.
6. Sarah Klemm RDN, CD, LDN, "Nutrition Tips to Promote Wound Healing," Academy of Nutrition and Dietetics, November 9, 2021, https://www.eatright.org/health/wellness/preventing-illness/nutrition-tips-to-promote-wound-healing.
7. "Improving Blood Flow to Speed Up Wound Healing," Advanced Tissue, June 11, 2015. Accessed on August 8, 2024, from the Internet Archive, https://web.archive.org/web/20210302174914/https://advancedtissue.com/2015/06/improving-blood-flow-to-speed-up-wound-healing/.

20. The Brain

1. R. Peters, "Ageing and the Brain," National Institutes of Health, National Library of Medicine, National Center for Biotechnology Information, February 2006, https://www.ncbi.nlm.nih.gov/pmc/articles/PMC2596698/.
2. "How The Aging Brain Affects Thinking," National Institutes of Health, National Institute on Aging, accessed May 20, 2021, https://www.nia.nih.gov/health/how-aging-brain-affects-thinking.

Notes

3. "How The Aging Brain Affects Thinking," National Institutes of Health, National Institute on Aging.
4. NIH/National Institute of Neurological Disorders and Stroke, "Scientists Monitor Brains Replaying Memories in Real Time," ScienceDaily, March 5, 2020, www.sciencedaily.com/releases/2020/03/200305203531.htm.
5. University of Tokyo, "Forgetfulness Might Depend on Time of Day," ScienceDaily, December 18, 2019, https://www.sciencedaily.com/releases/2019/12/191218090152.htm.
6. Jonathan Graff-Radford, MD, "Sundowning: Late-Day Confusion," Mayo Clinic, March 26, 2024, https://www.mayoclinic.org/diseases-conditions/alzheimers-disease/expert-answers/sundowning/faq-20058511.
7. "Alzheimer's: Can an Amino Acid Help to Restore Memories?," CNRS (French National Center for Scientific Research), March 3, 2020, https://www.cnrs.fr/en/press/alzheimers-can-amino-acid-help-restore-memories.
8. NIH/National Institute of Neurological Disorders and Stroke, "Scientists Monitor Brains Replaying Memories in Real Time."
9. University of Virginia Health System, "Brain Discovery Could Block Aging's Terrible Toll on the Mind," EurekAlert!, July 25, 2018, https://www.eurekalert.org/news-releases/474617.
10. BEC Crew, "Marijuana Compound Removes Toxic Alzheimer's Protein from the Brain," ScienceAlert, May 26, 2018, https://www.sciencealert.com/marijuana-compound-thc-removes-toxic-alzheimer-protein-from-brain.
11. Dennis Douda, "Mayo Clinic Minute: Is Alzheimer's Type 3 Diabetes?," Mayo Clinic News Network, November 7, 2017, https://newsnetwork.mayoclinic.org/discussion/mayo-clinic-minute-is-alzheimers-type-3-diabetes/.
12. Douda, "Mayo Clinic Minute: Is Alzheimer's Type 3 Diabetes?"
13. Elaine K. Howley, "Brain Fog: Causes and Treatments," *US News*, May 31, 2019, https://health.usnews.com/health-care/patient-advice/articles/brain-fog-potential-causes-and-treatment.
14. Dana G. Smith, "At What Age Does Our Ability to Learn a New Language Like a Native Speaker Disappear?," Scientific American, May 4, 2018, https://www.scientificamerican.com/article/at-what

Notes

-age-does-our-ability-to-learn-a-new-language-like-a-native-speaker-disappear/.

15. Erin Brodwin and Skye Gould, "The Ages You're the Smartest at Everything Throughout Your Life," *Business Insider*, July 31, 2017, https://www.businessinsider.com/smartest-age-for-everything-math-vocabulary-memory-2017-7.
16. Brodwin and Gould, "The Ages You're the Smartest at Everything Throughout Your Life."
17. Brodwin and Gould, "The Ages You're the Smartest at Everything Throughout Your Life."
18. Smith, "At What Age Does Our Ability to Learn a New Language Like a Native Speaker Disappear?"
19. Alexa Erickson, "These Are the Ages You're Best at Everything, According to Science," *Readers Digest*, April 28, 2021, https://www.rd.com/list/best-ages-in-life/.
20. Charles Patrick Davis MD, PhD, "Aging: The Surprises of Getting Older," On Health, February 26, 2018, accessed May 20, 2021, https://www.onhealth.com/content/1/surprises_aging_getting_older.
21. Rachel Wu and Carla Strickland-Hughes, "Think You're Too Old to Learn New Tricks?," *Scientific American*, July 17, 2019, https://blogs.scientificamerican.com/observations/think-youre-too-old-to-learn-new-tricks/.
22. Wu and Strickland-Hughes, "Think You're Too Old to Learn New Tricks?"
23. John Anderer, "Physics Offers Explanation to Why Time Flies as We Get Older," *Study Finds*, January 20, 2022, https://www.studyfinds.org/days-gone-by-physics-offers-explanation-to-why-time-flies-as-we-get-older/.
24. Anderer, "Physics Offers Explanation to Why Time Flies as We Get Older."

21. Dehydration

1. SaVanna Shoemaker, MS, RDN, LD, "12 Simple Ways to Drink More Water," Healthline, February 10, 2023, https://www.healthline.com/nutrition/how-to-drink-more-water.
2. "Dehydration and Stroke: How Are They Connected?," Michigan Neurology Associates. Accessed on August 9, 2024, from the Internet Archive,

Notes

https://web.archive.org/web/20230405025812/https://www.michiganneurologyassociates.com/blog/dehydration-and-stroke-how-are-they-connected.

3. Joji Inamasu et al., "Clinical Characteristics of Stroke Occurring in the Toilet: Are Older Adults More Vulnerable?," *Geriatrics & Gerontology International* 18, no. 2 (February 2018): 250–55, https://doi.org/10.1111/ggi.13168.

4. American Heart Association, "Dehydration Linked to Worsening Stroke Conditions," ScienceDaily, February 15, 2015, https://www.sciencedaily.com/releases/2015/02/150212092731.htm.

5. "Dehydration and Stroke: How Are They Connected?," Michigan Neurology Associates.

6. "Dehydration and Stroke: How Are They Connected?," Michigan Neurology Associates.

7. Shoemaker, "12 Simple Ways to Drink More Water."

8. "10 Reasons Why Hydration Is Important," The National Council on Aging, September 23, 2021, accessed November 15, 2022, https://www.ncoa.org/article/10-reasons-why-hydration-is-important.

22. What Is Diet?

1. Nicole M. Avena, Pedro Rada, and Bartley G. Hoebel, "Evidence for Sugar Addiction: Behavioral and Neurochemical Effects of Intermittent, Excessive Sugar Intake," *Neuroscience and Biobehavioral Reviews* 32, no. 1 (2008): 20–39, https://www.ncbi.nlm.nih.gov/pmc/articles/PMC2235907/.

2. "The Scary New Research on Sugar & How They Made You Addicted to It! Jessie Inchauspé | E243," *The Diary of a CEO*, May 1, 2023, https://www.youtube.com/watch?v=DnEJrgc1BCk. For more information on sugar and misinformation, see also Thomas DeLauer, "22 Most Dangerous Foods for High Blood Sugar | Jessie Inchauspé," May 15, 2023, https://www.youtube.com/watch?v=rt8YYdvox-Q; Dr. Bobby Price, "12 US Foods BANNED in Other Countries," May 31, 2023, https://www.youtube.com/watch?v=KDzTeCbDwII&t=8s.

3. "Student-Faculty Research Suggests Oreos Can Be Compared to Drugs of Abuse in Lab Rats," Connecticut College, October 15, 2013. Accessed on August 12, 2024, from the Internet Archive, https://web.archive.org/web/20240418032913/https://www.conncoll.edu/news

Notes

/news-archive/2013/student-faculty-research-suggests-oreos-can-be-compared-to-drugs-of-abuse-in-lab-rats.html.

4. "The Sweet Danger of Sugar," Harvard Health Publishing, Harvard Medical School, January 6, 2022, https://www.health.harvard.edu/heart-health/the-sweet-danger-of-sugar.

5. "Facts About Sugar and Sugar Substitutes," Johns Hopkins Medicine, accessed September 20, 2023, https://www.hopkinsmedicine.org/health/wellness-and-prevention/facts-about-sugar-and-sugar-substitutes.

6. "Substitutes for Sugar: What to Try and What to Limit," Cleveland Clinic, June 14, 2023, https://health.clevelandclinic.org/best-and-worst-sugar-substitutes/.

7. "Substitutes for Sugar: What to Try and What to Limit," Cleveland Clinic.

8. "Facts About Sugar and Sugar Substitutes," Johns Hopkins Medicine.

9. Camila Domonoske, "50 Years Ago, Sugar Industry Quietly Paid Scientists to Point Blame at Fat," *NPR*, September 13, 2016, https://www.npr.org/sections/thetwo-way/2016/09/13/493739074/50-years-ago-sugar-industry-quietly-paid-scientists-to-point-blame-at-fat.

10. PragerU, "Why Celebrity Trainer Vinnie Tortorich Is a Carnivore | Real Talk," June 9, 2023, https://www.youtube.com/watch?v=SYq2ORN9VJc.

11. PragerU, "Why Celebrity Trainer Vinnie Tortorich Is a Carnivore | Real Talk."

12. PragerU, "Why Celebrity Trainer Vinnie Tortorich Is a Carnivore | Real Talk."

13. "How Do Lobbying Groups Affect the American Diet," National Exercise and Sports Trainers Association (NESTA), May 7, 2019, https://www.nestacertified.com/how-lobbying-affects-dietary-guidelines/.

14. Bambi Turner, "Is American Wheat Different Than European Wheat?," HowStuffWorks, April 19, 2021, https://recipes.howstuffworks.com/is-american-wheat-different-than-european-wheat.htm.

15. "The Scary New Research on Sugar & How They Made You Addicted to It!"

16. Kris Gunnars, BSc, "22 High Fiber Foods You Should Eat," Healthline, May 3, 2023, https://www.healthline.com/nutrition/22-high-fiber-foods.

17. Isadora Baum, "Your Body's Protein Requirements Change Significantly as You Age—but How?," Well+Good, March 8, 2024, https://www.wellandgood.com/protein-requirements-by-age/.
18. Jillian Kubala, MS, RD, and Kris Gunnars, BSc, "16 Delicious High Protein Foods," Healthline, October 18, 2023, https://www.healthline.com/nutrition/high-protein-foods.
19. Rachael Link, MS, RD, "11 Best Healthy Fats for Your Body," Dr. Axe, June 8, 2024, https://draxe.com/nutrition/healthy-fats/.
20. Link, "11 Best Healthy Fats for Your Body."
21. Kris Gunnars, BSc, "Are Vegetable and Seed Oils Bad for Your Health?," Healthline, June 9, 2023, https://www.healthline.com/nutrition/are-vegetable-and-seed-oils-bad.
22. Kelsey Kunik, RDN, and Lauren Panoff, MPH, RD, "4 Healthier Cooking Oils (and 4 to Avoid)," Healthline, October 24, 2023, https://www.healthline.com/nutrition/healthy-cooking-oils.
23. "The Man Who Can Predict How Long You Have Left to Live (to the Nearest Month): Gary Brecka | E225," *The Diary of a CEO*, February 27, 2023, https://www.youtube.com/watch?v=r3atRG5wvtg.
24. "The Man Who Can Predict How Long You Have Left to Live (to the Nearest Month): Gary Brecka | E225."

Summary

1. Wenpeng You et al., "Total Meat Intake Is Associated with Life Expectancy: A Cross-Sectional Data Analysis of 175 Contemporary Populations," *International Journal of General Medicine* 15 (February 1, 2022): 1833–51, https://doi.org/10.2147/ijgm.s333004.
2. *The Longevity Film*, directed by Kale Brock (Sidney, Australia: Brock Creative Media, 2019).
3. Brock, *The Longevity Film*.
4. Brock, *The Longevity Film*.
5. Brock, *The Longevity Film*.
6. Brock, *The Longevity Film*.
7. Brock, *The Longevity Film*.
8. "The Man Who Can Predict How Long You Have Left to Live (to the Nearest Month): Gary Brecka | E225."

9. Becky Upham, "6 Unexpected Benefits You'll Be Happy to Know About Menopause," Everyday Health, May 23, 2023, https://www.everydayhealth.com/menopause-pictures/positives-of-menopause.aspx.
10. Jamie Ducharme, "This Is the Age When Your Self-Esteem Is Highest," *TIME*, August 22, 2018, https://time.com/5373095/self-esteem-highest-study/.
11. Rick Marshall, "The Origins of 11 Famous Star Trek Lines," Mental Floss, November 6, 2015, https://www.mentalfloss.com/article/50607/origins-11-famous-star-trek-lines.

www.ingramcontent.com/pod-product-compliance
Lightning Source LLC
Chambersburg PA
CBHW050555170426
43201CB00011B/1700